IN THE COUNTRY
OF ILLNESS

IN THE COUNTRY OF ILLNESS

Comfort and Advice for the Journey

by

ROBERT LIPSYTE

Alfred A. Knopf   New York   1998

THIS IS A BORZOI BOOK
PUBLISHED BY ALFRED A. KNOPF, INC.

Copyright © 1998 by Robert Lipsyte
All rights reserved under International and Pan-American
Copyright Conventions. Published in the United States by
Alfred A. Knopf, Inc., New York, and simultaneously in
Canada by Random House of Canada Limited, Toronto.
Distributed by Random House, Inc., New York.

www.randomhouse.com

Library of Congress Cataloging-in-Publication Data
Lipsyte, Robert.
In the country of illness: comfort and advice for the journey /
by Robert Lipsyte. — 1st ed.
p.   cm.
ISBN 0-679-43182-9 (alk. paper)
1. Catastrophic illness.   2. Sick—Psychology.   3. Medical
care—United States.   I. Title.
R726.5.L57   1998
362.1—dc21   97-31245
CIP

Manufactured in the United States of America
First Edition

For all my fellow travelers,
safe home.

Everyone who is born holds dual citizenship, in the kingdom of the well and in the kingdom of the sick. Although we all prefer to use only the good passport, sooner or later each of us is obliged, at least for a spell, to identify ourselves as citizens of that other place.

SUSAN SONTAG,
Illness as Metaphor

Contents

IN THE COUNTRY
OF ILLNESS

INTRODUCTION
Why Not Me?

I OFTEN BELIEVE that my travels in the country of illness have made me a stronger, wiser, better person.

And sometimes I think they have just been a string of bad trips.

The reality is probably somewhere in between, and I hope there is enough of it in these adventures and tips of a seasoned traveler to help you on your own journeys. That's all I am, a seasoned traveler—no traditional medical training, no knowledge of alternative remedies, no metaphysical secrets. But this I know: When we are sick or taking care of someone who is sick, we feel as though we are suddenly outside the borders of what we consider everyday life, and in another place. I call that place Malady.

Malady is another country, scary and strange. Its borderline is only one microbe, a rogue cell, an accident away.

When we are scared, feeling out of control, feeling like a unit on a conveyor belt of the medical-industrial complex, grateful for the casual mercies of doctors, nurses, technicians, aides, and receptionists, and confused by the rearranged relationships with friends and family members, it is easy to imagine being in a foreign land trying to learn the language and customs, calculate the currency, and remember the landmarks—all the while suffering ill effects from the local water.

From a distance, this kingdom of the sick seems to be an

aberrational place, a hateful, twilight-zone country off the charts, the kind of distant land that ancient mariners feared as abounding with monsters. So foreign, yet so near. But it's a real place with real people, and sooner or later we all get there.

Once we've survived a major trip to Malady, been seriously sick and recovered, we want to think we have learned something from such an absorbing, frightening, expensive, potentially fatal adventure. We want to believe that being sick has taken us deeper into ourselves, given us the strength to make some hard but necessary decisions, to love well and wisely, certainly to set better priorities, at the very least to stop sweating the small stuff.

I certainly felt that way. At the age of forty, having never been seriously ill, I rushed into Malady on a deluxe package tour, three weeks in the Memorial Sloan-Kettering Cancer Center, two operations and a two-year course of chemotherapy. I was scarred and I was scared, but I wanted to believe I had been enriched, enhanced, had become a better husband, father, brother, son, writer, for having taken that journey. Well, I certainly had more to write about, although I wince at the bravado still shouldering through my sentences, the puns, metaphors, and overreaching references that evoke an often pathetic need to remind myself and others that I might be down but I am still functioning, still trying to make my mark, if not some order, here. It is graffiti on the sickroom wall.

This book is also a work in progress; I still travel in and out of Malady, for myself and others. I have learned a great deal about the medical system and about the techniques of survival from my mother's long-term struggle to keep her diabetes under control and from the health problems of friends—Roger's kidney dialysis and transplant, Godie's Crohn's disease, Doc Sheehan's prostate cancer, Susie's progressive neuromuscular condition—as well as the stories of multiple sclerosis, Canavan's disease, heart attacks, strokes, AIDS, and Parkinson's disease I covered as a reporter.

My personal experience is mostly with cancer. Even though cancer is more than 100 different diseases, some of which are more treatable and less life-changing than the illnesses just mentioned, the word alone seems to have a terrible, almost mystical power; it can scare off friends and family, it can depress a patient out of all proportion to immediate danger, it can isolate you in Malady just when you need more helping hands. Because of my own experience, I feel a common bond with all patients and caregivers, especially in this turbulent time when the way we have become accustomed to receiving health care is undergoing seismic shifts. But then, so much is changing. My oldest friend, a gastroenterologist, was grumbling recently that he is now no longer considered a doctor; he is "a health-care provider." I said that I could sympathize, having just done some on-line work for my newspaper's new media department, where I was not considered a writer; I was "a content provider."

I began to find my voice for this book when Carey Winfrey took over *American Health* magazine in 1991. He wondered if I would like to write for it. Over lunch, we conceived a column—he named it "Close Encounters"—that would follow a middle-aged everyperson's search for health. It wouldn't be self-consciously traditional or New Agey; it could range from aspirin to yoga, from surgeons to shrinks. Before we parted that day, he laughed and said, "At your age, Bob, things will happen to you. You'll always have something to write about."

Big joke. Two weeks before my first column was due, I called him with the good news—I was going for a battery of tests. I might have cancer again. He was cool enough to commiserate and be delighted at the same time. "I'm sorry to hear that," he said, "but I *was* worried about that first column." Editors.

As it turned out, I did have cancer again, but the doctors missed it for most of that first year of the column, which gave me the chance to also explore dental surgery, sex, fitness, and a possible heart murmur. Most important, those four years of writing "Close Encounters" forced an introspection that did not come easily to me. I tend to plunge on through life, from encounter to encounter, without close examination. In writing the column, I thought seriously about manhood and courage. I saw how my life during wellness dictated my approach to illness, and how traveling through Malady was an education for my entire life.

But it was my father's first illness, at ninety, that made me really think about where I had been and what I had learned. Here was a man who had always made quick, don't-look-back decisions. Now Dad was suddenly at a loss to think his way through the choices that the doctors threw at him. My father, who has taught me so much, who has always been a major hero and role model, turned to me for advice. What did I really know? Still, I went with Dad into Malady. That trip became a warm-up to a journey with my former wife, Marjorie, that was one of the most profound experiences of my life. I've learned a lot, some of it useful, I hope. I've also learned to see the dark side, and I think that can be useful to you, too.

And somewhere along the way, I finally understood a joke I first heard in junior high school.

Guy goes to the doctor, worried sick. "Doc, every time I lean over my eyes bulge, my ears ring, and I start to choke. Sometimes I pass out."

Doctor examines him, gives him every test, finally says, "Sorry, but there's only one thing it can be, and it's fatal. You've got six months to live."

Guy takes all his money out of the bank, sells all his possessions, books a round-the-world cruise. Just before he leaves, he goes to a fancy store, buys shoes, suits, silk underwear. He tells the salesman, "I want a dozen of your best shirts, size-fifteen neck."

Salesman measures him anyway. "Sixteen neck."

"But I've always worn fifteen."

"Suit yourself. But when you lean over, your eyes'll bulge, your ears'll ring, and you'll start to choke. Some people even pass out."

When I first heard the joke, I thought it was very funny and was about stupid patients. When I was a patient myself for the first time, I thought it was sort of funny, and was about know-it-all doctors.

Nowadays, I don't think it's funny at all, and I know it's about the changing relationship between the patient who does not know the language or customs of Malady and the doctor who has no time and/or inclination to teach. In these days of managed medical minutes, how would the doctor know about a tight collar? The doctor sees the patient naked and knows nothing more about the patient than what the machines print out. There is far less time available to take the detailed history that can assure a future.

Being sick doesn't make me an expert on medicine, although spending most of my lifetime figuring out this one dumb joke has been an education I want to pass on. I hope I can be a helpful guide to Malady, that this book will answer some questions and raise some. I also hope you will come to my way of thinking that there is one question you need never ask: "Why me?"

There may be a technical answer—a rogue cell, a misshapen chromosome, a marauding virus, a toxic chemical— but there is no cosmic philosophical answer, certainly not "Because you needed it" or "Because you deserved it" or even "Because you can take it." That's just blaming the patient.

If we were born to die, we were also hard-wired to get sick, even briefly, along the way. Why not me? is as good a non-answer as any. Reynolds Price, a writer who survived spinal cancer, says that the real question should be, "What's next?"

So, skip the philosophy and prepare for the journey.

PART ONE

Innocents Abroad

I

MY OWN JOURNEY began with a vague ache in my right testicle, which seemed larger and firmer than usual. I began touching my right testicle every so often to check if the swelling had gone away and it became a habit, a tic. In the beginning, I would touch it only when I happened to be in a bathroom, but soon I made visits purely for self-exams. So many journeys to Malady seem to start this way, undramatic distant warnings, a tingle in a joint, shortness of breath, a fleeting chest pain after running for a train.

When I couldn't keep my hands off myself—poking through my pants pocket on the street, at the swim club, at the dinner table—and when I was giving Margie hourly updates, like testicular weather reports, it seemed time to go to our local family doctor, a pleasant technician we usually visited for strep throat cultures. Probably nothing, we agreed.

On my calendar, under June 20, 1978, I wrote the doctor's name and "Balls." It was my first attempt at tumor humor, which would soon become very important.

As it turned out, the doctor was not concerned, so I didn't have to be. Normally, after I'd been standing awhile, blood vessels called varioceles would drop down into my scrotum like strands of linguine and sometimes feel twingey. For twenty years doctors had told me not to worry about it, although I did. This was probably a variation, the doctor said.

He called it "an unspecified inflammation" and prescribed tetracycline for two weeks. He told me to take hot baths several times a day and to put my feet up whenever I could so the varioceles could slide back up into my body. It was non-alarming advice, yet proactive; I was doing something to correct a minor problem. I stopped touching myself more than a few times a day. The ache kept nagging for the next two weeks, but at a greater distance. Because I had faith in the doctor's nondiagnosis—you bet I wanted to believe it—the anxious edge that often stimulates pain faded.

(This was the same doctor who prescribed Provera for Margie's painful menstrual periods. Perhaps, she later thought, it was a cause of her own cancer.)

I was feeling physically fit that summer. I was forty years old, a husband, father, suburban householder. My weight, a chronic problem, was down to 174, only five or six pounds more than it should be. I was swimming and playing tennis almost every day. I was traveling to the South Bronx regularly to work on the local political campaign of a friend, and the tough, streety Puerto Ricans I was hanging out with were turning up as characters in a not-very-thrilling thriller I was writing about a fortyish, novel-writing journalist whose life was turned upside down by a female journalism student who challenged him to be better. Based on guess who?

When I went back to the family doctor, he shook his head in puzzlement and sent me up the medical chain to a local urologist, who thought my swelling was "epididymitis," an inflammation of a tiny tube of ducts attached to the testicle. He prescribed ampicillin and Chymoral and longer, hotter sitz baths. This was July 17.

If it's not epididymitis, I asked, what could it be? He shrugged. I asked him one of the three most common dramatic questions (the other two are, "Is he dead?" and "Are you having an affair?"), and he shook his head. At forty, he explained, I was too old for testicular cancer, a disease of men twenty years younger. Come back in two weeks if the swelling doesn't go down, which it should, he said.

Margie remembered those weeks, more poignantly than I do, as my vain attempt to poach the swelling away. She described me sitting in the bathtub, twice a day, with books, music, once even, she said, with a cigar in a show of bravado. I don't remember the cigar, and my calendars never mention baths. But I'm sure she was right. Who wants to remember something so pathetic?

I do remember during those weeks that Fraidy, the little white kitten that my daughter Susannah and I rescued from her Brownie leader's car engine, had to go to the vet, and that my son Sam took two fastballs on the same finger during two different Little League games. The second time, as I remember it, he hit a home run off his finger, but broke it. (Sam remembers that he struck out.) I remember that Margie and I took the kids to camp in the Adirondacks, that we visited them, and sat through the camp production of *Annie*, in which the role of President Roosevelt's Secretary of Labor, Frances Perkins, was played by a boy. Margie talked about that most of the way home. Perkins was the first female Cabinet member! What kind of camp were we entrusting the kids to? I remember that we saw movies, *Coming Home* and *House Calls* and *An Unmarried Woman,* met friends, and almost every afternoon after writing we drove to the local swim club and did laps.

What I didn't remember for a long time was my mounting concern, the rising certainty that something was wrong. Another vignette that Margie remembered and I had erased, or at least buried deep in the hard drive, was the pool party at which I asked my oldest friend, Mark Chapman, a gastroenterologist at Mt. Sinai hospital, to feel my swollen testicle. He lived in the next town, and one night at his house, after the guests went inside for dinner, I made him follow me into his pool house. I pulled down my trunks. Obviously, I was getting scared. He said it was probably nothing to worry about, but of course I should check it out right away.

On the last day of July, I returned to the local urologist. Margie came with me this time, and followed me right into his examining room. This was not routinely done in 1978. She was ahead of her time. Also, she told me years later, she thought I "looked tortured" and was "a basket case," atypically passive and weak. The urologist was surprised by Margie's presence, but probably intimidated. When he tried to at least draw a curtain, she said she had seen me naked before.

After he examined me, he suggested "we take a look-see" at what he now called "a testicular mass." As he explained it, the look-see was a simple operation called an orchiectomy. A slit would be cut in my groin near the hair line, and the testicle lifted out by the long duct cord that connected it to the rest of my body. Dangling like a yo-yo on the end of its string, the testicle would be examined. If it was benign, it would be dropped back into the sac. If it was malignant, the string would be snipped and the testicle would be examined further to determine the next steps.

When I asked why he didn't take the easy route through the sac to the testicle, the same way he would go in for a vasectomy, he explained that should it actually be cancer, malignant cells could spill and spread. He didn't tell me that most testicular masses turn out to be cancerous.

Margie asked, "How many of these do you do a year?" It was her first cancer question, the first of thousands, and it still stands as one of the best. When it comes to any kind of important decision or procedure, it is essential that the doctor be experienced. Never, ever, hesitate to ask about experience and credentials.

The urologist admitted that he and his suburban partners got to see only two or three cases like this a year. We sensed he looked forward to it as a good experience for the team. He never suggested we go to a larger center with more experienced doctors.

We made an appointment to have the operation at a local hospital in a week. (This doctor disappears from the story now, but my memories of him are still warm; months later, he actually called me to find out what had happened and how things had turned out. The fact that he cared enough to follow up, even if it was only professional curiosity, makes him unusual and a good guy in my book.)

I was scared. It was not The Dread, that cloak of catatonia I would feel later when I knew more, but it was enough to dry my mouth and loosen my bowels and leave me staring into the future, unable to make the next move. I crossed my legs just thinking about the orchiectomy. I had always been terrified of a hernia operation, and at a time when vasectomies were becoming popular I rejected having one out of the fear of being cut down there. And here we were about to go to a hospital for what might turn out to be a serious disease. I was, according to Margie, a "whimpering wreck."

She kicked me into gear, ordering me to get advice from some of those pre-meds with whom I'd gone to college. They were now doctors in major teaching centers. Mark was away on vacation, and so was Arthur Rifkin, a psychiatrist, but Dave Kinne, a leading breast surgeon at the Memorial Sloan-Kettering Cancer Center, was at work. I was lucky, though even more scared now; to an inexperienced patient like myself, that world-famous cancer treatment center conjured up more visions of illness and death than of health and healing. As a sportswriter, I knew that Babe Ruth had died there.

Steady, kindly Dave took my call very seriously. He told me to wait fifteen minutes, so he could call first, then to call Poppy, the secretary of the great Dr. Willet F. Whitmore, Jr., who would give me the first available appointment. That turned out to be for the next morning. I relaxed a little, feeling an expert was on the case now.

I took the kids—Sam was ten, Susannah seven-and-a-half—to see *Grease*. We ate at a local pizza joint. I usually loved such kid-stuff outings. But I was distracted: I kept jostling my testicle during the movie and the meal, expecting the swelling to go down before morning and embarrass me in front of Dr. Whitmore for making such a fuss.

It was still there when Margie and the kids dropped me off at Memorial on their way to the airport to pick up visiting cousins. After my appointment, I would catch a bus back home in time for the welcoming barbecue.

Dr. Whitmore turned out to be the ur-urologist, the famous surgeon who had treated writer Cornelius Ryan and former Vice President Hubert Humphrey. He was a handsome, middle-aged swashbuckler who swept into the chilly little examining room with his young resident as if they were Batman and Robin. The moment I saw them, my fears vanished; Whitmore managed to create an unreal world in which we were setting off together on an adventure. Terry and the Pirates! Captain Midnight! I had nothing to worry about.

They smiled knowingly as they took my history, cupped and squeezed my testicle as they examined it. No doubt about it. They seemed energized that I would give them another go with the enemy.

Dr. Whitmore said, "Looks suspicious to me; let's go in there. We should do this right away."

I was so caught up in his spirit, I said, "What are you doing this afternoon?"

Surgeon and Robin winked at each other and clapped my shoulders. I was pleased to imagine them thinking what a gamer I was; this boy has come to play! That tendency to want to please our doctors is a dicey matter. When it leads us to become active in our own healing, to take better care of ourselves, it's terrific, but when it makes us passive, too accepting, it's dangerous; a lot depends on the doctor, of course, and a little skepticism on our part never hurts. In this particular case, my wanting to please the doctors was probably helpful. It carried me mindlessly through what would have been anxious hours.

Dr. Whitmore told me to go out and have a second breakfast, as if I'd been able to have a first, buy a toothbrush, then call Poppy, who by then would have made arrangements for my admittance that very day. There would be a day of tests, he said, then the orchiectomy on Friday. I might be able to go home by Sunday. I left the examining room as if it were a locker room—if not overjoyed, at least up for the game.

It was my first professional contact with jock surgeons, who are different from other doctors, more like quarterbacks, test pilots, hot street cops, those give-me-the-ball types who seem to subscribe to the macho creed of If in Doubt, Do Something! The scalpel is a performing tool in a win-lose game, a life-and-death theater, and the surgeon is the star, surrounded by supporting players. Other specialists are often more important than the surgeons, but none can beat them for sheer glamour.

Many surgeons are too quick to cut, true, and their optimism is frequently unjustified. The way they coo over a fresh cut—"That looks so gooood!"—or reverently touch fading surgical scars calls for satire. Unless, of course, those cuts and scars are on your body and the surgeons are leaning over you as if you are the game they've just finished playing. Not quite so funny. And when things go wrong, surgeons, like athletes, tend to place blame beyond themselves, on the referees, the field conditions, the stubborn refusal of the patient to heal properly. But with the big game on the line, nothing is as encouraging as the hearty confidence of those jock surgeons who think they can carve you to victory. Their confidence is not always well placed, but it is always welcome.

. . .

MY ROOM, 831, was pleasant and light. The first two nights I shared it with a shrunken, pearl-gray man whose curtain was drawn most of the time. His visitors seemed to be his wife and their grown children. They looked grim, especially during whispery bedside conferences with doctors. In the middle of the second night there was chatter and scuffle—I was tranquilized and I remembered it as a dream—and the next morning the curtain was open and his side of the room was uninhabited. Even the plastic water jug with the bent straw was gone. His mattress was rolled to the foot of the bed. The nurses would not tell me where he had gone. I later found out that a rolled mattress in the morning meant the guest had checked out that night. Permanently.

The first operation, the orchiectomy, less than forty-eight hours after Whitmore first hefted my testicle, was no big deal in retrospect, although the hours around it—my first overnight in a hospital since losing my tonsils at four—were vivid. Everything was freighted with significance, alarming, confusing. I was in-country now.

There was a bewildering, eventually annoying, parade of man-child doctors marching importantly into my room with big steel clipboards and little black notebooks. They were tired because they were overworked and they were defensive because they weren't quite sure what they were doing. The youngest were the worst, hiding their studenthood behind the slightly distracted arrogance then in vogue at better medical schools.

This being early August, many were just rotating into urology, or on urology fellowships that had begun in June. They were practicing their interviewing, chart-scanning, testicle-squeezing. On me. I had no way of reading their "Hmmmmms" and "Ah-hahs." What do you see, I asked, is it bad? They had no information for me because they didn't know much yet, and they had yet to develop the lofty benevolence of their elders. So they hmm'd some more, and left me sweating. Had I known more then, I would have been able to disregard their murmurings, let them poke and move on or even send them packing. It was not likely any of them could help me. The downside of a great teaching hospital is all the eager students.

Meanwhile, the nurses were bucking me up with the false chirpiness of flight attendants in a wind shear. I didn't know how to read that, either. Were they so cheerful because I was in such bad shape?

And then there were the aides, clanging bedpans in the night. Practicing the cymbals for Carnegie Hall? For the Urologists' Ball?

Thank goodness for tumor humor.

We didn't have a name for it yet (the first time I saw that term in print was in a 1980 Young Adult novel, *Waiting for Johnny Miracle*, by Alice Bach), but that Thursday night before the first operation, we had our first experience with that enormously helpful genre of sick humor.

Tumor humor is not warm and friendly; it does not necessarily release feel-good endorphins. It is not what the writers Joseph Heller and Norman Cousins have prescribed, and it is not the "Laughter Is the Best Medicine" feature my grandfather used to read to me from *Reader's Digest*. Tumor humor is scrappy and sometimes nasty and tasteless, a sort of chemotherapy for the spirit, necessary and never nice. Trash talk. Really sick jokes.

Example: Margie sat on my bed and while we were going over the next morning's procedure for the hundredth time, I suddenly asked, "So if they pull it out and it's cancerous, what do they do with it after they test it? You can't just throw a malignant testicle in the garbage disposal, can you?"

Soon we spun off into a dark fantasy about my diseased testicle floating off into the world. I mean, after all, what *did* they do with the cancerous testicles they threw away? Into the sewer, out to the ocean, adventures on other continents? Did people pick them up, display them as found art?

This probably doesn't seem all that funny to you. As I read it now, it doesn't seem all that funny to me. But I remember how hilarious it seemed then, not because of its intrinsic humor, but because it gave us some release and it also gave us some sense, however false, of control. We might be swept away on this tidal wave, but we still had an oar in the water. We could still crack wise.

Tumor humor is a tough sell until you need it. And then it's a saver. Tumor humor is for the comedian, not the audience. I learned that when a friend of mine, suffering from prostate cancer, had a heart attack. I was taken aback when he said, "See, I told you guys that cancer wasn't going to get me." His recovery might be in part attributable to that attitude, which keeps you positive and aggressive in the pursuit of getting better.

Tumor humor is a form of gallows humor, the brave and edgy, often self-mocking jokes that the oppressed, the minority, the scared silly tell each other to keep from crying.

Two Jews about to be shot by a firing squad. Abe says, "Wait a minute, what about my last request? I want a cigarette." Izzie elbows him and whispers, "Don't make trouble."

Or

Down South in the sixties, Dick Gregory is about to tear into a whole fried chicken when those three brothers Ku, Klux, and Klan walk into the restaurant and say, "Boy, whatever you do to that chicken we'll do to you."

So Gregory kisses the chicken's butt.

Get it?

Cancer has no special claim on tumor humor. It should be

practiced by every traveler in Malady. In recent years, some of the best examples of that gallant, life-affirming whistling in the dark have come from AIDS patients. But it is tricky, since it can seem offensive if it comes from people who haven't earned the right to use it—by being a patient or a caregiver—and it shouldn't be used by patients and caregivers to shut out others who might be helpful. No rules here. I just remember how it helped get us through that night before the first operation. We were able to make believe everything was normal. After all, weren't we being our usual smart-alecky selves?

After Margie left, a wiry young man named Edward strutted into the room and shaved my pubic area with entertaining theatrics. He told me he had never lost a patient, and that this was a simple deal. He made me feel good until he said, "Good luck," in the same tone Las Vegas changemakers use when they give you rolls of coins for the slot machines. I didn't know then that everyone says "Good luck"—it means only as much as you want it to mean—but I worried about it until my sleeping pill hit. Actually, I hated to take that pill and stalled as long as I could; it meant letting go, losing control. This, I later found out, is very common. But unless you plan to stay up during the operation and direct it, take the pill. Get your rest.

There was a lot of bustle the next morning. Margie was there as I was wheeled out of my room. I remember saying, "I'm sorry," to her. I really was sorry, anticipating all the anguish and dislocation I was causing her and others. We talked about it later because she was touched that I could have such a feeling at that time. It was probably a good thing, in that I wasn't totally absorbed in my own immediate concerns, but if it led to my becoming depressed over something that was not my fault it would clearly hamper recovery. It's worth keeping in mind.

I think I saw Dr. Whitmore, but everything was mostly dim and pale and chilly. I woke up in Recovery, shivering, one of many slabs of meat on tables lined along a wall. Nurses moved among us. I must have been in better shape than most of the patients coming out of the operating rooms because I looked around, noticed a woman's pretty face, and studied the outline of her body under the sheet.

That I could appreciate the good-looking woman on the next slab, though only theoretically, indicated to me that I was sort of okay. But I was very cold, bone-chilled, and for years I wondered if that was from the shock of the cutting or the anesthesia. Or was it from the temperature of the operating room, presumably kept cold for good medical reasons, perhaps to slow the blood or kill off the bad germs.

It was almost twenty years later that I read an article explaining that operating rooms were routinely kept at about 65 degrees so that the surgeons, heavily gowned and sweating under the bright lights, could perform in comfort. According to the article, a new study had found that patients who were kept warm during an operation, even with something as simple as a blanket, recovered more quickly and had far less risk of infection than those operated on in a cool room. A drop in temperature interferes with the body's defense against germs. Finally, hospitals are turning up the heat.

I was still too groggy to be scared when I was told the next day that I had cancer, and that it looked as though it had broken out of the testicle. One of the doctors said, "It's a bad one," but his tone seemed to indicate that this would be less a danger to me than an exhilarating challenge for him.

Dave Kinne told Margie that it would be several days before "the numbers were in." It sounded like off-track betting to me. There would be more tests, and a second, much more extensive, operation.

I'd be in-country for a while.

2

THE EIGHTH FLOOR of Sloan-Kettering was the Gettysburg of Urology, an entire floor dedicated to the deadly civil wars of the genito-urinary system. Most eighth-floor patients were men and, not to stretch this military metaphor too fine, we all wore the same uniforms—those silly blue gowns tied in the back with our bottoms hanging out. Being regimented by disease was helpful. There was an instant support network, a chance to share information and rumors and, of course, to discuss the doctors, nurses, aides (that side wore green or white) on our own terms.

I was on my feet pretty quickly after the orchiectomy, an operation not much more involved than fixing a hernia. In fact, hernia was going to be the cover story, conspired Margie and I, at least until I found out how serious all this was and figured out what kind of game face to wear for the outside world. I didn't want to wear the scarlet C on my forehead, the wrong varsity letter for a freelance writer who wants to sign long-term contracts.

The compulsion for secrecy, tough on Margie fielding routine calls at home and certainly antithetical to her open nature (her announcement to an afternoon crowd at the swim club, a booming "Bob has cancer!" without preamble or hello, has become a family classic), did not last long. In fact, in a sharp turn, I decided that I was going to become Captain

Cancer and liberate my brother urological patients with the same brave honesty Betty Rollin had shown in her 1976 bestseller, *First, You Cry.* Because AIDS has come to overshadow most cancers, it's easy to forget just how out-there and in-your-face was Rollin's book and subsequent interviews. She made jokes about cancer! While some people thought she might have trivialized the life-threatening aspects (in one famous scene in the book, Rollin shops for a button that could serve as a false nipple under clothing), there was no question that she had thrown open the topic to frank, useful discussion.

I talked to a friend, Neal Conan, who was a producer and correspondent at National Public Radio, about broadcasting from bedside, maybe even talking my way through the second operation. Live or die, I said, we will make public radio history with a real-life series, a cancer opera.

Neal was encouraging but noncommittal, which was exactly what I needed to stay up while that wild high subsided and I settled into surviving in my corner of the medical-industrial complex, a gulag cum boarding school where you make your friends and create your new life. The only model I had for this was the six months I spent on active duty in the Army Reserve, especially the two months of basic training. I didn't keep regular notes until the end of the tour when I was safely ensconced in an information office, writing press releases about heroic cooks in the mess halls of New Jersey. But it was one of those experiences you don't forget.

In 1961, at twenty-three, soon after the draft deferment for married men was canceled, I joined an Army reserve unit. I was halfway through a five-year first marriage that had begun to end before it began. And so there was a certain cold comfort in being shipped off to the sandbox of Fort Dix, several hours down the New Jersey Turnpike from my Manhattan home. By that time, I was four years out of college and a *New York Times* sports reporter, which was not going to impress sergeants who had fought on Pork Chop Hill in Korea or the gung-ho upstate farm boys whose first pair of real dress shoes was Army issue. If I was going to be much of a man, I'd have to prove it among men, who have a different, perhaps slacker, standard of manhood than do women. I'm still not completely sure of this, but I sense that most adult females demand a certain level of responsibility, of restraint, of grown-up behavior—the best word is the Yiddish *mensch*—before awarding boys the stripes of a man. Males are satisfied by loyalty, physical courage, and good fellowship, which is particularly easy to achieve on sports teams and in the Army.

So even though I hated the Army for the loss of my freedom and the waste of my time, I enjoyed the fun of shooting guns and camping out and narrowing the worries of life with a group of like-minded pals. A simple life. I made intense Army friends, and we bonded against the sergeants, the officers, and the system itself. Sometimes we even railed against the Cold War and the political diseases of history that had brought us all together.

Like a sports team manipulated by control-freak coaches, we were whipped into shape by the macho sergeants, who were always sneering that we recruits weren't "man enough" for what they would make us do. They intimidated us physically and emotionally—there were unanswered daily challenges to step out behind the barracks and fight, there were Kotexes left on bunks. We responded by trying to please them, even if it meant selling out each other. We also responded by challenging one another's manhood, constantly calling each other "fag" and "queer." (In my limited corporate experience, I've learned that all this gets smoother, but never better, in the civilian work world.)

The fat city boy who smashed his own nose with a rifle butt to avoid a twenty-mile march was labeled a "pussy" by the sergeants, who suggested that we beat the shit out of him.

After all, the sergeants said, if he can get away with this now, can you imagine what he will do in combat when you depend on him to cover your back? When we did nothing about it, there were extra nights of cleaning up offices and picking butts off the ballfields.

Ultimately, it was what we did for one another, often in defiance of the Army's regulations and the sergeants' manipulations, that created the bonds among us. We helped our clumsy, even our lazy, brothers clean their rifles and boots, we encouraged the unfit to climb the obstacles, we drilled the stupid before tests. I was not a particularly skillful soldier, merely adequate on my best days at crawling, shooting, setting up a tent, or spit-shining, and I got a lot of help along the way. In return, as the top pen of my clerk-typist class, I pulled a few semiliterates to graduation in my wake. Most men did what they could. And those who didn't reach out, unless they were contemptible, dangerous sleazeballs, were usually forgiven; men learn to give slack because they want to be sure it's there when they need it.

The Army was the first place I saw real kindness among men. It was okay to show compassion, even an almost tender, "feminine" caring, for a buddy who had sprained an ankle, ripped open an arm on barbed wire, received a Dear John letter, lost a weekend pass. Of course, the moment the crisis was over, you could mock him again, reveal his secrets to the squad, try to beat him at cards, beer-drinking, chippie-chasing.

Seventeen years later, those months at Dix seemed like training for another kind of hitch.

MY SECOND Memorial roommate, Greg, was about twenty, a lean, wiry laborer, with the powerful but asymmetrical muscles you get from real work rather than working out. He had Popeye forearms and a sunken chest. He also had the thousand-yard cancer stare. He could lie on his bed for hours boring a hole in the ceiling with his eyes. I've done it myself and, depending on what's going on deep in your head, it is either very destructive or a harmless time-killer.

Greg didn't want to talk much, but it's hard for a journalist to respect that, even in the cancer ward. After a while, he told me that he'd had an accident at work in which some building materials had slammed into his groin. The company had tried to avoid responsibility, and by the time Greg finally got serious attention at a local hospital his testicle was the size of a softball. He wasn't sure if the accident had been a lucky one that alerted doctors to the cancer, or had actually caused the cancer. The doctors didn't have a definite opinion, or at least didn't give him one.

Greg's first operation had been performed in the local hospital—the doctors were excited because they didn't get to see too many testiculars. There was some concern now that their inexperience had allowed cancerous cells to spill free.

His mother and sisters bustled in and out with cookies and cakes Greg never ate. His depression was profound. They offered the food to me, and I helped them out. Alas, not even cancer spoiled my appetite.

Greg's father looked like his son, lean and wiry, but weathered. He wore clean, ironed work clothes, matching blue pants and shirts. His name, which I never could make out, was stitched over one pocket. He would sit for hours in a chair at the foot of Greg's bed staring at Greg staring at the ceiling. Sometimes his eyes would redden and brim with tears, and he would hurry out for a smoke in the visitors' lounge (this was 1978; they even smoked on the lung cancer floor). Greg and his father hardly ever talked, sometimes watched a ballgame. I imagined that the father wished it had happened to him instead of his boy, that somehow he was trying to absorb the bad cells or give energy. Sometimes I felt worse for him than I did for Greg. When my own kids were babies, I was a cradle-kicker, constantly assuring myself that they were only sleeping, and I can still remember how powerless I felt when they were sick and in pain. Susannah's chicken pox once had me near tears. It was not hard to imagine how Greg's dad felt. When children are sick, there is always the problem of dealing with the anguish and even guilt of parents without letting it get in the way of caring for the real patient.

In 831, we were often joined by Danny, who was as blabbery and soft as Greg was silent and hard. He had thick, wavy, jet-black hair, and full red lips. He looked like a Holiday Inn piano man. He came to talk. He started telling his story as he walked into our room the first day. Between Greg's cookies and my questions, 831 became the unofficial day room for the young testicular set. We tumor-humorists called it the Make-Believe Ballroom, after a popular radio disk jockey show of that time.

Danny had squeaked through high school and flunked out of a local community college. He lost some jobs because he wouldn't "take shit," he said. Finally, through a cousin who was "connected," Danny got a job in a gambling casino. He turned out to be a Phi Beta Kappa in dealer school. He had found something he could do well. He rented a swinging bachelor's pad, which his mother flew out to decorate. He bought a muscle car and some cool clothes. He had ladies lined up. He was studly.

He was showering one evening before taking a "real classy lady" to dinner and a show when he felt the pea on his testicle. He was terrified and after a flurry of phone calls home he flew back to New York. His folks took over; a local hospital, the orchiectomy, a diagnosis of malignancy, and here he was, waiting for Memorial to review all his tests and give him some new ones and figure out what to do next.

What with Danny blabbering and Greg staring and Bob trying to be wise but flip, we were three standard characters in a foxhole waiting for orders to do or die. We were soon joined by the squad sergeant, the most gallant of us all, a blue-collar businessman named Alec who was defiantly optimistic despite test results that clearly showed he was the sickest in the group, which made him our leader. When the four of us and any other testiculars we could round up got together at Greg's bakery, we sounded like a cross between soldiers waiting for battle and young docs discussing the literature. All travelers in Malady talk the talk pretty quickly. We had the basics down cold.

Testicular was fairly rare, accounting for only about 1 percent of cancers in men, cropping up in about 6,000 Americans a year (although the men were mostly young, non-Hispanic white men, which gave it some research urgency for doctors of that time). There were three main types of testicular cancer—seminoma, embryonal carcinoma, and choriocarcinoma. Each was classified, through surgical biopsy, blood tests, and X-rays, into three main stages.

In Stage I, the cancer cells were still in the gonad. In Stage II, they had started trekking up the retroperitoneal lymph node trail, which is located below the diaphragm in the back of the abdominal cavity. In Stage III, the cells had metastasized and broken for the lungs, liver, and brain, where testicular can get nasty and in some cases (about 5 percent) even deadly.

The diagnosis to get was Stage I seminoma, although I never met anyone who had it. Early seminoma can be blown away after the orchiectomy with radiation, without a second operation. Sergeant Alec believed that Stage I seminoma did not exist, that it was a false hope held out to keep us from jumping out a window between discovery and diagnosis.

If the maybe-mythical Stage I seminoma was the cancer of

choice, Stage III chorio, what Alec had, was the worst. He would need massive doses of the toxic cisplatin, which could turn you deaf and shut down your kidneys. We were all grateful cisplatin existed, and in conversation with civilians carefully called it a "powerful medicine" rather than a "toxic drug," to spare them fear spasms. But among ourselves we used the toughest language we could, being members of a very dangerous gang, perhaps a commando unit, despite our flimsy gowns flapping open at the bottom. Actually, we were endangered more than dangerous, though not as endangered as most of the other patients on that urological eighth floor, who were older and sicker, with bladder and prostate cancers. But we were in much better shape to posture and bond. We were also much luckier.

Ten years earlier, the "cure rate" for most testiculars had been only about 10 percent. Cure in this case meant the patient was alive five years after diagnosis. (If you died in the sixth year, and this is still standard for all cancers, you would probably be counted twice, once as some doctor's Win, once as some doctor's Loss.) By the late seventies, because of the new chemotherapy drugs and progressive surgeons such as Whitmore who did not believe that men could be saved by the knife alone, the rate was edging toward 90 percent.

I had the middle cancer, embryonal (although my records note traces of seminoma, chorio, and "mature" teratomas), and it was in the middle stage.

In the week between the orchiectomy and the big operation, the retroperitoneal node dissection, I hung out with the ballteam, as we also sometimes called ourselves in the tumor humor mode, and took an endless series of tests, which I came to look forward to as breaks in a long day. It was amazing how soon the hospital floor became my reality and procedures that once would have made me squirm just to hear about became interesting to undergo. I remember my fascination with the lymphangiography, in which dye was injected into my right foot so an X-ray could track it through my body. A few months earlier, just the thought of such a procedure would have actually made me dizzy; I'd been known to get lightheaded, have to sit down fast, after one of my kids got bloody. Paper cuts made me sway. Now I looked forward to invasive stunts.

The lymphangiography was performed in one of Memorial's many dank little basement rooms. I leaned forward in a wheelchair and enjoyed the show. Once the area was numbed, a little hole was cut between my first and second toes, then a tube was inserted and the dye pumped in. Naturally, I had to prove I wasn't out of the loop by making a few smart remarks—"Ahh, a tasty dye, dry and fruity," was a typical example. Truly stupid medtechs or those with attitude might scowl or blink, but most would chuckle indulgently. They seemed to tolerate faux feistiness, sometimes understand and even encourage it, at least as well as most nurses did, and far better than most doctors. As a practical matter, a patient who can psych himself up is less likely to freak out, certainly will be easier to deal with. From a patient's point of view, at least from mine, feeling part of the action allayed fear.

The medtechs who ran the X-ray machines and administered the minor procedures tended to have up-tempo personalities. They were mostly youngish; lately, in New York, more of them seem to be black and Hispanic men who keep up an easy, calming chatter. The East Indian, Asian, and Russian blood-takers seem a little more reserved. Like pupils studying teachers and prisoners studying guards, patients study health-care pros—their power, however brief, seems absolute. When one ignores you, rattles you around, or yells at you for not producing easy veins to puncture, the sense of vulnerability can be overwhelming. The foreignness of Malady, when you don't know what is being done to you or why, can be confusing and frightening. Asking questions in a friendly way, inserting yourself into the procedure without challenging anyone's professionalism (unless, of course, something is going wrong), may be the best way to dispel that sense of dislocation. The medtechs, of course, have parents, children, siblings, uncles and aunts, too, and once they see you as members of the human family, their approach softens, becomes less rote. Talk music, sports, clothes, weather, if you can. You may or may not actually get better technical care, but you may feel less anxious about the care you do get. That's worth a lot in Malady.

Visitors to Room 831 sometimes enhanced the sense of foreignness by their own awkwardness and anxiety. For starters, most of them either lowered their voices (so as not to rouse the demons of disease?) or feigned that hospital heartiness—"You look great, Bob, you can't be sick, you're on vacation, you're hiding out, you don't want to finish that book . . ."—that sucks the air out of your lungs.

You want to be treated seriously—though not always *that* seriously—and you don't want your illness trivialized. You want to choose who makes the jokes, when, and what they are. You want people to *listen* to you, to respond to your moods, to let you lead the dance. If you want to play Pollyanna or play Terminal Man, it's your call.

This is tough because the visitors are also scared, for you and for themselves, and they may be less traveled in Malady than you are. Sometimes you want them to go charging out to the nurses' station and scream for a long-awaited painkiller, or go buy cookies so the night nurse will drop into the room more often, or just shut up about what a dump you've picked. You've got to tell them what to do.

I quickly learned to keep visitors to a minimum for a number of reasons, some of them questionable. The least defensible reason was not wanting to be seen in a position of powerlessness, the macho man laid low. I wanted to think of myself as still capable of telling people to take a hike, or even to get up and leave myself. I hadn't yet learned how other people can help you heal. When I'm sick I prefer to be left alone, to curl up in a ball. I learned that from my father.

The best reason to keep visitors to a minimum was that I didn't want to expend energy I needed for myself; after my family and a few close friends, I couldn't be singing and dancing for all the people who needed to be assured that I wouldn't die before their flowers did. That energy is a critical factor in your getting well, and it is not selfish to conserve it.

Margie thought I was going to die, at first. I never thought so. I believed the doctors who told me that the cure rate was better than 90 percent. More important, I was *inside* the battle, absorbed by the busy-ness of hospital life, by the social aspects, by the struggle to come back from operations, pains, fears.

Margie, despite caring for the kids, running the household, and driving back and forth from the suburbs, had more time to think and less new information. She had grown up in the thirties and forties, when polio was the clear and present danger and cancer was the beast in the corner that could only be mentioned in whispers, lest it wake up. People in the neighborhood were "*very* sick," the italics in the voice along with a shrug, a raised eyebrow, a frown, making it clear that "the Big C" had struck again. One wouldn't have been surprised if the newspaper obits had referred to "c-ncer" as if it were sent by "G-d"; they compromised with "after a long illness."

People who had cancer died in those days. Their cancers were diagnosed too late, and there were fewer aggressive, effective therapies. They wasted away. And because it was somehow shameful to have this crab clawing through your body, nobody talked about it. Patients, "for their own good," weren't told they had cancer. Doctors thought the diagnosis would kill them even before the disease did. You could talk about your heart disease, but not your cancer.

Something else people didn't talk about, and that took us a little by surprise, was how any major illness can rearrange family relationships. Children grow up in a hurry taking care of parents disabled by strokes or lupus or heart disease, and the mutual dependencies of spouses are changed when one of them gets sick. Driving back and forth in the almost nightly thunderstorms of that August, Margie screamed and cried and got stronger. I had been the driver in the family; now she was driving under terrible circumstances. She was in charge. Even if I didn't die right away, she assumed I would be diminished and she would have to do double duty. To use that political-sounding term, Margie was "empowered" by my illness. This was a positive aspect of a negative experience, made even more positive when I neither died nor became a shell of myself. This "empowering" happens a lot, and it should be expected and welcomed, although patients often resent it as a side effect of their illness. The most famous examples of this came in the wake of Vietnam, when American soldiers returned home after years as prisoners of war to find "the little woman" had taken charge. Many of those marriages didn't survive.

MY PARENTS, then in their seventies, were typically supportive, although they were upset. My father, who except for a hernia operation had never been sick or hospitalized, was stoic and a little distant. He seemed to be denying that I was sick. But he was right there, offering help. Margie remembers him pressing cash into her hand. He knew there would be many little out-of-pocket expenses, he said, and he wanted to relieve that pressure. It was a generous and welcomed act. If you know people well enough to give money in a natural, graceful way, do it. If it's offered, take it. There are always extra costs, and giving money, like doing chores, watching children and pets, and driving, is just another way of helping out in a crisis.

We were lucky that I was covered at the time by Writers Guild of America health insurance. I had written a screenplay, and while the producer had typically tried to avoid paying for my benefits, the Guild had chased him down, in the nick of time. Even then, health insurance was a major worry. These days it often seems a more critical problem than the disease itself. More on this later.

My mother, who had undergone considerable doctoring, including several major abdominal operations, tried to keep her hand in, dispensing advice and second-guessing doctors and nurses, but her heart wasn't in it. This was cancer, after all. She, too, was intimidated by the word. Later, during a brief period in which I became interested in a possible direct cause of the cancer (there had been reports of men with testicular cancer whose mothers had taken DES early in pregnancy), she became strangely evasive. I also remembered a series of shots as a small kid; the doctor had Mom practice on an orange before she began injecting me at home. What were they for? Were they hormones? She couldn't remember. Was there a connection? Did it matter now? I lost interest after a while. I decided that unless getting the answers would alter my treatment—which the doctors did not think was likely—there wasn't much point in making Mom feel guilty. My parents felt bad enough.

The entire family rallied. My sister, Gale, was researching alternative therapies because Margie was prepared to take me to German spas for a cure if all failed here. Sam, then a beefy ten-year-old who could be passed off as a smallish fifteen-year-old (the minimum age to visit the cancer floors unless you had your own tumor), was grown-up yet jolly on his visits. I talked to Susannah on the phone. At seven, she was obviously too young to come up. I'm sure keeping children out is good for the sanity of the staff and for general health and hygiene, but both patients and their kids can benefit from some kind of supervised visits. Children wouldn't feel so abandoned and it would help patients feel connected to the everyday world to which they are trying to return.

Friends, especially doctor friends put off by Memorial's no-nonsense jock briskness, almost a mood of enlightened car repair ("You got it bad, we fix it good" should have been their motto), seemed most uncomfortable. My friend Mark was appalled at the Memorial bedside manner. But I liked the Memorial approach. I saved an index card on which I recorded some lines from Graham Greene's *The Human Factor* on August 5, the day after the orchiectomy.

He found himself again an object on a conveyor belt which moved him to a destined end with no responsibility, to anyone or anything, even to his own body. Everything would be looked after for better or worse by somebody else. Somebody with the highest professional qualifications.

While I wasn't quite willing to turn myself over completely, there was a great deal of comfort in not fighting the system. The time had always passed more easily in the Army when I let my mind become olive drab, too. The worst times in the Army were re-entering the barracks after a weekend pass, still stimulated by the sounds and sights of freedom.

During the three weeks I was in Memorial, two books of mine came out, the paperback version of a young adult novel, *One Fat Summer,* and a hardcover memoir of me and the champ, *Free To Be Muhammad Ali*. I kept them hidden in my drawer. I didn't want that part of my life on display here. I didn't want to answer questions. How could this happen to you? You've published books! Some weird pride perhaps; cancer was still shameful.

Or maybe it was the special resonance of those two books. The semiautobiographical *One Fat Summer* was about Bobby Marks, a fourteen-year-old who loses almost forty pounds during one tumultuous school vacation. It was the furthest I had ever gone in revealing myself. I had plunged back into the prison of my fat to capture the feelings of being an outsider because of my size. Being fat had been a kind of illness, perhaps a rehearsal for cancer.

Free To Be Muhammad Ali was about my professional coming of age. The *Times* had sent me to cover Cassius Clay's first championship fight because the primary boxing writer, like most of his generation, was disdainful of this loudmouth kid. In 1964, this Little Richard with a punch appealed mostly to the young and nontraditional sportswriters. When he won, he became my front-page story. He kicked off my career.

Bobby Marks and Muhammad Ali would return in wondrous ways to give me comfort later on. I didn't want them exposed in the cancer ward just yet.

My testicular pals knew I was some kind of a writer, but since none of them was any kind of a reader, the discussion always began and ended with the line, "You could write a book about this place." If I had thought I really would, I would have taken far more notes than I did. But for some reason I wanted to live that experience, sink deep into it, absorb it honestly rather than keep it at a distance by pretending it was a journalistic assignment. So much of my life has been secondhand, I thought; this is very real stuff and I want to be present as performer, not scribe.

. . .

WHEN WE MET each morning after breakfast, at least one of us would be absent, for an operation, a test, a lousy stay-in-bed day, and more than one of us would be in pain. We gave each other a lot of the slack and unself-conscious tenderness I had seen in the Army. There was still competition, though muted, and a pecking order existed—Alec was the leader by virtue of being more cancerous as well as having a top-dog personality and rangy cowboy looks.

So we listened patiently to Danny's whining until it threatened to swamp us and then Alec would buck him up; we stared at the ceiling with Greg; we suffered Bob's scared sarcasm; we pretended to believe that Alec had had sex with his wife, in his hospital bed, the day after his orchiectomy. His wife happened to be very pretty and nice and hot—her sexuality cut through even that place—but she also seemed sensible enough not to have excited Alec while his stitches were still oozy.

Actually, sexuality was the one topic we never discussed honestly and the one we desperately needed to know more about. The younger men were very concerned about the effect that the operations and chemo might have on their procreational and recreational sex lives. There was no psychological counseling, and other than the recommendation that we freeze sperm, invariably given too late to create a viable bank, there was little information from the doctors.

While we might gossip about doctors and nurses, like schoolkids about their teachers, we never found out anything. But the aura of male power in the hospital in those days was implicit. There were few female doctors, certainly I saw none on the urology floor, and the relationship between doctor and nurse at a place like Memorial was potentiated (a favorite word about drugs) by the combination of job, gender, and class. In a major-league international teaching center in a big city, the doctors and nurses tend not to travel in the same social circles, as they might in the community hospital of a smaller city.

I was lucky never to have gotten caught in those days in one of the nasty little flare-ups between nurse and doctor that I encountered later. My case seemed to be straightforward enough, the medication standard. I might notice a dismissive grunt or two by a doctor toward a nurse, and a nurse's sneer and eyeroll at his retreating back, but that was all. There were, of course, civil wars. But we all knew enough never to get caught up in whatever was going on, be it love or hate, even if we had our own feelings about a doctor or nurse. That's a good general rule. You will be leaving Malady someday, and the nurses and doctors know they are staying and will have to work out their relationships. Stay out of it. You can offer friendship and support to someone, but unless your care is affected, mind your own business.

A few years later, a friend, a doctor at a leading teaching hospital, felt the iron claw of a heart attack in his chest one evening as he was leaving work. He took a deep breath on the steps, made his diagnosis, and plunged on, to the New York City subway, then to a commuter railroad. Some ninety rush-hour minutes later, when his wife picked him up at their suburban train station, he calmly told her to drive him to the local hospital.

When he related the story to me a few nights later in his hospital room, I asked the obvious question. He sat up in his bed in a cheery, modern, semiprivate room and gestured toward a hall filled with smiling nurses. "Back at my place," he said, "they would have killed me."

Back at his place, or Memorial, the younger nurses typically lived packed in nearby high-rises or out in the boroughs, while the doctors had fine suburban homes or smart Upper East Side apartments. When they did get together, it was usually for some recreational, extramarital sex. Even the jock surgeons, many of whom had actually been athletes in school, tended to be catching up on sex; years of serious studying in college and medical school had crimped their sex lives. Even the non-jock types were suddenly sex objects. How all of this affected patient care, I don't know. It could have distracted them or it could have stimulated their desire to do good work. The nineties' TV medical dramas offered both answers.

It was clear, though, that the doctors were either not sensitive to our need to know how our sexual equipment would perform after orchiectomy and beyond, or they didn't know themselves. They acted as if even discussing it was irrelevant to their primary mission, to save lives. In fact, it wasn't until a research Fellow showed up to do a study on impotence that we got to ask some questions. There still weren't satisfactory answers. In the course of the retroperitoneal node dissection, we were told, nerves affecting potency and sperm delivery could be damaged. How often did that happen? Was it permanent? Orgasms might feel different. In what way? He didn't really know.

(This research Fellow, thirtyish, friendly and chubby, made enough of an impression for me to write down his name in my scanty hospital notes. Harry Reiss. I described him as very smart, needing a shave, willing to listen, and needing to tuck in his shirttail. He was different enough from his snappy, know-it-all colleagues to lead me to imagine he would either become a leading researcher in the field or go begging for referrals. And then I pretty much forgot about him for twenty years. Forgive the suspense; we'll get back to him later.)

So we didn't talk about future sex and we fell back on our tumor humor. We babbled about "blackballing" guys we didn't like, and we rated the staff with balls instead of stars. Whitmore got four balls, the max, while the night nurse, who seemed to enjoy waking patients by dropping a pan or kicking the bed, got one half of one ball, the minimum.

We also entertained one another with real-life campfire stories, some of which were probably true. Danny had great Mafia tales from his father's old neighborhood and from the casinos, a few of which I realized I had read in books by Gay Talese and Mario Puzo. Alec had construction tales that made building a suburban shopping center sound like the Seabees carving landing strips out of the jungle in World War II. Even Greg might chip in with a vignette about the characters who collected the garbage and put out fires in his hometown. I told about sports figures I had interviewed ("What's Yogi Berra *really* like?").

But the story that really captured the group was about the Cancer Man, a character who had caught my imagination although I did not completely believe he existed.

In the early sixties, I had written a *New York Times Magazine* article about two city narcotics detectives who were on their way to setting all-time records for arrests and for kilos seized. Their street names were Bullets and Cloudy. They were convinced that the local Mafia and the international drug exporters had hired a famous assassin, known as the Cancer Man, to take them out.

There was no way he would fail, they would tell me during the long stretches of downtime at wiretaps or on surveillance. The Cancer Man, diagnosed years before with an incurable malignancy, was credited with most of the world's high-level, unsolved criminal executions. Besides his street smarts, skill with weapons, and nondescript looks, he had no fear—he was already sentenced to death. In fact, the incredible chances he took might be attributed less to nerves of steel than to his death wish—he would rather die quickly in a hail of slugs than slowly in bed.

(You can imagine how we chewed on that one in Room 831, although we never quite got around to talking seriously about suicide.)

Bullets and Cloudy felt their only hope was to outlast the

Cancer Man (he was backlogged with contracts, he was that good), but they never took special precautions. It added to their romantic edge. That and their disregard for other people's rights in the battle against drugs made their company exciting, fascinating, and eventually disgusting. After my magazine piece appeared, which they liked, they told me that they were on the verge of a really big heroin bust that would make them world-famous, and me, too, if I played my cards right. I could write their book. This was very heady stuff for me at twenty-four, especially when I actually got a book contract. But we eventually fell out, and I returned my book advance, which led the surprised publisher to offer my name to Dick Gregory, whose autobiography, *Nigger,* I eventually did write. Meanwhile, it turned out that Bullets and Cloudy were not kidding about the big bust. Eddie Egan became an actor and film consultant before he died in 1995, and Sonny Grosso is a successful TV producer. Their big case was called "The French Connection."

At this point in the story, my pals, most of whom had seen the 1971 movie if they hadn't read the best-seller, rolled their eyes and hooted and groaned. Well, everybody blows some deal, they would say, and comfort me. We could also laugh about it. It wasn't cancer. I think it was Danny who said I should try to find the Cancer Man; he would make an even better book. When he busted out of this joint, Danny promised, he would check with his sources and get back to me.

I'm still waiting. But I have also never stopped daydreaming about the Cancer Man, and wondering if I would use a terminal diagnosis as a license to kill.

THE SECOND operation, the retroperitoneal node dissection to chart the extent of the cancer's spread, was going to be an eight-hour exploration during which I would be split open from stem to sternum so Whitmore and his surgical Fellow, the improbably named Dick Chopp, could rummage elbow-deep inside me, tallying lymph nodes invaded by cancer cells. That would determine future treatment. It was Chopp, a prairie preppie who looked as though he had just walked off a midwestern golf course, who told me, "The cancer is caught now because you were on the ball, no pun intended."

There was a stream of docs, nurses, and techs the night before that operation. I remember the anesthesiologist, a Brit named Archie, who seemed smugly pleased to tell me what a "mayjaw" operation this was and how he would be "teddibly" busy keeping my fluids in balance as the surgeons "handled" my bowels. It would take at least twenty-four hours for me to recover, he said, and for three days afterward I could expect to "be out of it, and you would prefer it that way, to be sure." Not being all that sophisticated, I didn't realize just how important Archie was. For all their flash, the surgeons aren't the only ones in the operating room; the specialist who balances your blood and gases is worth checking out too.

Then Edward strutted in to shave me. My lucky charm. He had never lost a patient, right? He was flattered that I remembered his name, and he told me that Whitmore was the best.

"He lost Hubert Humphrey," I said.

Edward recoiled. "Oh, no. Hubert waited twelve years. If he had come in on time he would be alive today."

After he left, I talked to Susannah on the phone, and she sang a song from *Annie*, "Tomorrow," in a sweet, quavery voice ("The sun'll come out, tomorrow . . ."). I tried to cry, I wanted to cry, it seemed as though I *should* cry, but I couldn't.

I finally did get to cry at Memorial, but like most everything else cancer-related (most everything else becomes cancer-related, a recurring problem), it didn't quite nick with anyone's theory or design. I didn't cry because I was scared or because I was in pain or because I was tough enough to be tender or because I was ashamed of the fix I had gotten my family into by getting sick. I cried in rage and frustration because I was thwarted. I couldn't fart.

But first, the operation. Years later, reading the record of it, I got the sense of how major it was, although I didn't fully understand what they did. It read like a Tom Clancy novel, lots of hardware jargon you don't understand but which sounds exciting. The inferior mesenteric artery was "sacrificed" and the interaortocaval chain was "attacked" and "small venous oozers and small arterial pumpers were tied." It was *The Hunt for Red October*, only the quarry was a rogue cell instead of a rogue sub. My transverse colon was laid on my chest. While they were rummaging around inside me, they did an appendectomy, which included a "purse-string suture," and my abdomen was closed "using an interrupted Tom Jones fashion closure." I didn't understand much of that the first time I read it, still don't, and am not sure I need to, although I do believe in getting your medical records, because you can always find someone to translate them if you need to know something. Just how different the language of Malady is from what I speak every day was made clear by this line in the record: "the patient tolerated the procedure well, and had no difficulty."

I would have written, "the patient was blissfully out cold and didn't start having a tough time until he woke up."

Margie had a tougher time; no one called her as promised, and she roamed hospital corridors that night barred from seeing me or finding out how I had done other than that I was still alive and in recovery. Maybe a small matter in retrospect, but not at the time. If there is any brief for managed care as far as patients are concerned, it might be the slim hope that competition will breed caring as a good business practice. If every HMO has the same machines, customer service may eventually become important as the margin of victory, for profit. This is certainly something for individual caregivers and patients' rights organizations to use as leverage; the awful anxiety of those hours is so easy to alleviate— even a telephone call with a nurse would be appreciated.

It was several days before I got my brains back and could wonder at the tubes snaking out of my nose and up my penis and into my arms and hands. That was when Chopp explained my diagnosis and prognosis. The cancer had traveled up into several lymph nodes, but he didn't think it had metastasized beyond them. There would be chemotherapy. I would be hearing from the chemotherapists, he said. Chopp admired the ugly railroad track of black stitches up my belly.

"Looks gooood," he cooed more than once. The jagged red wound would become a scar in forty days, at which time I could "test" it.

I asked Chopp the essential question: "Will I be able to run the marathon and play the violin?"

"I see no reason why not," he said, grandly.

"Great," I said. "I've never run a marathon or played the violin."

He smiled coldly and pinched my toe through the sheet, the surgeon's signal of patronizing affection, and swaggered out. I liked Chopp; his confidence in himself gave me confidence in my future, but I couldn't help having the subversive thought that he had learned the pinch and the swagger in med school.

Quickly, I learned not to offer such commentary to my floor buddies. It made them uneasy. My three closest pals were blue-collar guys, none of whom had doctors in their families, or socialized with doctors. They might have their own wry comments about individual doctors, even criticisms of the medical system, but it was always from a respectful distance. There was a certain awe of doctors' accomplishments and skills (how I felt about auto mechanics and sculptors) and an implicit acceptance of the order of things, with patients near the bottom, perhaps only above the women who brought the food trays and emptied the bedpans, sometimes in the same motion.

I had no such awe or acceptance. I grew up with doctors, dentists, and druggists in the family and I played in the homes of kids whose fathers were doctors. I had no illusions about them being a superior breed. I knew that doctors' wives paid for cars and summer camps in cash, usually in small bills skimmed from patients' fees and not reported to the IRS, and I overheard amusing dinner table talk about hypochondriacal patients who were paying for vacations and home repairs.

Of course, I also saw doctor dads leave the dinner table for long telephone consultations, rush out at night, agonize over the treatment of a patient in the hospital.

My first wife's uncle, in whose apartment we lived one summer, was a dermatologist who would never allow a procedure to interfere with a symphony concert. Margie grew up in the same house with another uncle who was a Veterans Administration doctor. He booked procedures around golf dates. Many of my high school and college friends became doctors and dentists, and while most of them entered the profession with idealism and a genuine wish to help people, they also assumed that their early expenses and hard work would entitle them to a comfortable and secure living. In the fifties and sixties, young doctors could be certain that "M.D." also meant "Much Dollars." It helps to keep in mind that most doctors are ordinary people with special skills they learned in a school. The skills didn't come as a divine gift. And we are their customers, their reason for working, not the lucky recipients of their munificence. Of course, when you find a great doctor, talented and humane, be properly grateful.

. . .

THREE DAYS after the operation, an Irish nurse named Sheila—I love her still—ordered me out of bed to take a shower.

"Okay now, let's get up," the good sergeant bellowed. "You smell like a billy goat."

"A shower?" I croaked. "I can't move. Besides, the bottles'll break." The IV fluids in those days were in glass bottles, not soft plastic bags.

"You think you'll cut yourself worse than that?" she asked, jerking a thumb at the *gooood* red track down my belly. "So I'll get you a Band-Aid. Now get up, it's a shame. How can I face your family letting you look and smell like this?"

She chased me into the bathroom and slammed the door. It was one of the most intense short experiences of my life. Was I in there half an hour, an hour? I moved very slowly, very carefully, thinking through each placement of a foot or a hand as if it were a chess move. I kept measuring the distance between the swaying glass bottles and the jutting tile corners of the shower door. The handicapped move this way, plotting their logistics as if they are storyboarding movie shots.

Slowly, carefully, with a mounting exhilaration, I shaved and showered. I came out knowing I could do anything I needed to do.

My next goal was to go downstairs to the coffee shop with my intravenous bottles hanging from a rolling stand and have lunch with Susannah. It became an obsession. But I wouldn't be allowed to leave the floor until the tube in my nose, which was attached to a wall unit and pumped toxins out of my stomach, was removed. And that wouldn't happen until I passed wind, proof that my bowels had returned to life. Movement, I was told, would stimulate the stomach activity, and eventually provoke the desired flatulence.

I put a deadline on my goal, a lunch date with Susannah in two days. Reasonable goals for patients are a good thing because they can focus your activity, give you something more specific to achieve than just "feeling better." You will get out of bed, you will spend a half day at work, you will take a trip, visit a friend. Since I needed to shake my innards into action, I stretched and twisted and walked laps around the floor, fourteen circuits of the oval corridor to the mile. Various members of the ballteam did laps with me and I sometimes walked with men recovering from bladder and prostate operations, but they moved a lot slower, spoke a different dialect, and were both jealous and contemptuous of my disease, which they called "the kind of cancer you should get if you have to get cancer." It always comes as a surprise, although it shouldn't by this time, that within every disease group there are further competing subgroups. How many of your arteries were clogged, ask the heart patients of each other? How high is your stump? Exactly what type of multiple sclerosis do you have? It's human nature, I guess, but sometimes I wish there were more camaraderie among the travelers in Malady.

The night before my lunch date, my stomach had not even growled. I picked up the pace. No one could keep up with me. As the shifts changed and the floor became quiet, nurses who'd sung out "You're going to make the Olympics!" began to roll their eyes and look away. This was a crazy man.

A resident suggested I take a break. I brushed him off and plunged on, round and round, past the bluish glows of TV sets through open doors, past mutters and moaning and now and then a call for help. I had to keep moving, I told myself, because I had to fart because I had to have lunch with Susannah because it would prove I was still connected to that world beyond Malady.

And then somewhere along the way, I forgot everything except that I had to keep moving. Round and round, mindlessly; by dawn I had no idea what I was doing or why.

I didn't quit and I didn't collapse, but sometime before breakfast someone just steered me into my room and let me fall on my bed. I lay there, face down, melting into the threadbare blanket, choking on the black tube. I had failed. I wouldn't see Susannah. I began to cry, whiny tears at first, then great convulsive racking sobs. My body shuddered. My face was drowning in salty water.

I struggled to get up, I wailed, and then an electric shock slammed me down. And I farted.

No question, my gut rumbled. When the resident put his stethoscope to my stomach, he smiled and pulled the tube out of my nose and I laughed.

I still smile when I think about it—what a happy story! Where else but in Malady could a fart seem so sweet? But where else but in Malady is an internal organ recital fit for a public audience? Anything goes that gets you through. Nothing is embarrassing or shameful as long as it is real. Be prepared when you go there, long-term resident, day-tripper, helper, visitor, to talk freely—and helpfully—about parts of the body that don't normally appear on your radar screen.

As for that lunch, I remember it vividly. I was not eating or drinking yet, and I sat with Margie, Sam, and Susannah at a table in the coffee shop, my IV fluids bubbling out of their bottles into tubes pinned into my hands. Susannah, so pretty and poised at seven and a half, looked up from her lunch at my pale bubbles and asked, "Are you having ginger ale, too?"

I almost cried again.

THE LAST FEW days in Memorial were almost pleasant. I was an old boy now, and I had a certain standing. I was a squad leader. Danny and Alec were gone. Greg was still there, staring. I wandered into other rooms looking for fellow testiculars. I liked to sit on a young newcomer's bed and reassure him and his parents (who were usually just a few years older than I) that Whitmore was an Ace, that Memorial was the Place. Just relax and concentrate on getting strong again. You only need one testicle.

I'd go up to the recreation lounge on the fifteenth floor, a sunny room with a little outdoor deck, browse the library, consider taking up block printing or découpage, listen to a Judy Collins wannabe sing, watch Zero Mostel in *The Producers*. It was a veritable cruise to nowhere except we were wearing turbans over bald skulls, dragging IV racks, missing major body parts.

Once, a young Hispanic in cut-off jeans under his gown who looked like one of the South Bronx guys I'd hung out with the month before came up in a wheelchair with a boom box blaring salsa, which I would have hated on the outside. I gave him a thumbs up; we are alive, my man, riddled with termites but still baaaad. I understood his need to re-create some semblance of his everyday in this foreign place. I could cut him slack.

That was my good side. I was just as happy to let the bad Bob out. One afternoon I went down to the cafeteria with Margie, and found myself a table away from a middle-aged man in street clothes smoking a fat black cigar, blowing thick noxious clouds my way. I started screaming at him, I went for him, bottles banging. Luckily, he jumped up and ran out. I've thought about that incident, and while I don't exactly cringe with shame and regret, I don't slap a gold star on my forehead either. Smoking was not a moral crime in those days, not even in a cancer hospital, and I think I let my righteousness out like a deranged Rottweiler. It did make me feel better, but who knows how that stogie was comforting him. Maybe he had a wife or child dying up-stairs.

And I can't honestly be rational about it, either. Emotional swings are common when you are sick, from the disease, the tensions, the drugs, the vibrations you may be getting from relationships changed by the situation. You may not always be able to control the swings, even to cope with them, but understand that they are yet another routine scenic stop on the Malady tour.

Otherwise, the last few days were calm. I would miss my friends, as well as Sheila and some of the other nurses, several of the doctors. I was getting stronger; I wasn't in great pain. Most of the time, a hospital stay is a transition between being ill and recovering. It isn't what we consider real life; its purpose is to get you back to real life, and so you think of yourself as in a state of grace, of relaxed rules. Hospital rules. Friends being extra nice. I was looking forward to being home, but even then I sensed that the real tests were to come.

The chemotherapists showed up a few days before I was discharged, an unlikely-looking team, the round, messy, bearded Davor Vugrin and his oncology Fellow, Tom Reynolds, a crew-cut thirty-two-year-old from Ohio. They capered around my bed, jabbering, interrupting each other. They were as different from the surgeons who had preened over my scar as artists are from jocks.

They explained that within two weeks I would begin a two-year course of outpatient chemotherapy. Exactly which chemicals, and their strengths, had yet to be determined. There were more tests to study. There were at least five protocols of chemo, from mini-VAB, the lightest, to VAB-5, the closest to an atomic blast. I would find out what the letters meant when I needed to. Yes, there might be hair loss, mouth sores, vomiting, fatigue. I asked about marijuana, then being used covertly to suppress nausea.

"We don't supply marijuana," said Dr. Vugrin, "but if they jail you we bail you."

He giggled at his joke. It seemed as though we were planning a vacation together.

I asked them the test question: "Will I be able to run the marathon and play the violin?"

Reynolds didn't miss a beat. "Your marathon times will be slower at first, because you'll want to stop to smell the flowers. The immediate improvement will be in the violin, where your icy technical brilliance will be joined by a new depth and compassion."

Then he laughed and danced out of the room. I couldn't wait to start chemo.

3

EVEN NOW, when people say to me, "You beat cancer," I have three reactions.

I knock wood. I say to myself, Nobody beats cancer. And I reply, "I beat chemo."

Recovering from major surgery is heroic in a traditional, storybook way, like recovering from a battle wound or an accident or, most common in current American storybooks, coming back to play after a sports injury, a knee wrecked while trying to score a touchdown or while trying to wreck someone else's knee. But as much pain as you have to suffer, as much as your head is clouded by anesthesia, as hard as you have to struggle to get joints and organs working again, it is a finite task with a precise goal—getting back in the game, back to everyday, ordinary life. You can feel proud of yourself for small achievements, even heroic on the installment plan, as you see incremental improvement. Everything is easier and better if you have people cheering you on, as I did. It is the opposite of chemo, which is more like grinding life, one day at a time.

Cancer patients, of course, aren't the only people who take drugs with unpleasant side effects, although we seem to get the major share of publicity. My friend Godie, who has taken the steroid prednisone in an attempt to avoid, or at least postpone, further surgery for Crohn's disease, reports nasty mood swings from that chemotherapeutic agent, along with unwelcome face and body changes. Godie has been a stoic exemplar in the stubborn way he has pushed himself through periods of pain since childhood. Godie sails on.

Crohn's is one of several incurable, although generally nonfatal, intestinal diseases that together affect an estimated two million Americans. These diseases often begin early in life and can have an enormous impact on long-term self-esteem, not to mention adolescent social and sexual development. Abdominal pain, rectal bleeding, and high fevers are common, and often sudden and uncontrollable. It's very hard to even think about the soccer team or the prom if you are never sure you'll get to the bathroom on time. And when the chemo drugs turn you moon-faced, it's hard to turn that face to a world that may not know what you are going through— especially hard if you are embarrassed by your disease. Cancer, in recent years, has become less shameful and more heroic; all diseases need similar public relations make-overs.

Start the campaign at chemo. The medical and self-help literature on chemotherapy generally tends to gloss it over, calling it drugs or medication, referring almost parenthetically to such possible side effects as nausea, hair loss, fatigue, mouth sores, in a low-key-enough way not to scare people away from potentially life-saving treatment.

Meanwhile, some chemo vets recall its horrors with the passion of incest survivors or traumatized soldiers. The battle scenes are vivid—the clumps of hair coming loose in your hand, the retching long after there is nothing left to vomit, the disgust at one's own swelling, wasting, twitching body. Put two of us chemo-heads together and you'll hear the pharmacological equivalent of the Battle of the Bulge being compared to Little Big Horn.

There's a history of discussing drugs from the extremes. Traditionally, dope is either, like cool, man, or the subject of reefer madness. The medical casualness toward chemo, a poison that goes after any fast-growing cell (which includes hair follicles and mucous membranes), is a disservice—and yet plenty of patients take an intravenous shot before breakfast and go off to work. On the other hand, Sergeant Alec nearly died from his chemo. It shut down his kidneys and put him into dialysis.

People who are unprepared for chemo think they are the only ones who have ever gone through such torture, and sometimes they quit. People scared off by chemo may be missing their best chance for recovery. Every so often there is a story about a youngster who runs away rather than take treatment. If there is a follow-up story, it is invariably about the kid's death.

Nobody tells the full truth, however, which is that at its worst, chemo is punishing and spirit-sapping and still may not make a difference in your prognosis. At its best, it's the nuisance that saves your life. You'll never know where your treatment falls between those poles until you try it. Still, it seems primitive to take poison to be saved.

The three weeks between discharge from Memorial and the start of chemo treatments, with Margie and the kids cheering me on, I could feel like a running back trying to get the ball again. Because I was in fairly good shape ("A well-nourished, well-developed Caucasian," according to the one sentence in my chart I totally understood), and getting excellent care and support, my progress was fairly rapid.

The first week home, however, if I sat in too soft a living room chair, ten-year-old Sam would have to pull me out. That was a sudden insight into the future—being sick as a kind of preparation for being old. I had to move slowly and carefully because my body was a weather map of pains, hotter, fiercer in some places, like my surgical scars, constant but low-level, in my spine and head. My bowels were not yet working regularly, which was common. Parts of me were still numb. My evacuation route was the body system I thought most about, which is why, I guess, they call old age the second childhood.

Years later, a big, athletic friend struggling with Hodgkins disease told me, "I have new appreciation for the elderly, their sense of vulnerability. At the newsstand yesterday, three youngsters were horsing around and almost slammed into me. A few months ago I would have grabbed them by the collars. Now I felt fragile and I just tried to get out of their way."

Soon after he told me that, I was in northern California and had the chance to try out two very different hotel bathrooms. In one, the bathtub could be entered only by clambering over a black marble ledge that was almost as high as my groin. When wet, it was treacherous. I ended up getting in by a method suggested in the writings of C. Everett Koop, the former Surgeon General. I sat down on the ledge, carefully swung one leg over at a time, then stood up in the tub and slowly lowered myself. It worked. I felt safe and in control. And old.

In the second hotel, I was put by happenstance in a room equipped for handicapped guests. The toilet was a little higher than I was used to, and the sink and the light switches were a little lower, but all the bars and handles made getting in and out of the tub easy. Again I felt safe and in control. And old. But old, I believe (with greater assurance every passing year), is a lot better than old and sick, or even just sick.

By the second week out of the hospital, I was walking to town a mile away and thinking of getting back to work on that breakthrough thriller. Margie had ordered a reclining chair, assuming my long convalescence sitting by a window, reading. She canceled it by the end of the first week. But we did end up buying the first VTR (pre-VCR) in the neighborhood, a big wooden RCA that served us well for many years. We never would have bought it (like my father, who waited my whole childhood for TV "to be perfected" before he bought a set, I was not about to jump on some fad) if I hadn't gotten cancer. The cancer gave me permission to splurge on a luxury item that turned out to be one of our real joys. We watched movies as a family and we taped shows for me to watch during days I was recovering from chemo. Every time we agonized over buying some appliance or taking a vacation, one of us would bring up that VTR. We needed a trip to Malady to make a purchase that gave us years of pleasure. Let that be a lesson. Do not postpone joy. My parents bought us an early black-and-white video camera that had to be plugged into the VTR. We wrote, directed, and shot little plays. More joy.

The blockbuster hit of Susannah's eighth birthday party was the instant replay of the party itself. The kids watched themselves for hours. The lesson was repeated more forcefully—do not defer healthful things that will give you pleasure. Don't wait for serious illness to give you permission. I wish I could say that I learned from that and was never a silly pinch-penny again. But once you get back to everyday life, you tend to be your old self again. After all, wasn't that the reason you wanted to get well?

Those first few weeks home I began to think this cancer stuff was a hype. I fell back on sports metaphor, not surprising for someone only seven years away from daily sportswriting. I began to think I was Ben Hogan coming back to golf after the car crash, Frank Gifford after the concussion, Joe Namath or Billie Jean King returning from knee surgery. Of course, nobody is ever as good again, but . . .

These days, I have jaundiced feelings about the epic heroism we attach to athletic injuries. My God, these jocks have the entire Mayo Clinic under the stands waiting to ER them, the best pain-killers, steroids for healing, top rehab specialists, all for free. Big deal for their heroics.

Of course, on the other hand, all this medical attention is not to get them well for a long, healthy life, but to get them back in the game. Ordinary life for them is the short-term goal of resuming short-term combat, where they will surely be hurt again. It is rare to meet a former athlete, particularly a pro football player, who can easily get up from a soft chair without at least wincing. Almost all of them live with pain forever. Unlike the accident victim or the surgical patient, however, the athlete made a Faustian bargain to live with pain in exchange for a glorious half-life—if, indeed, young athletes really have the knowledge to make an informed decision.

I knew all that then, but I was still happy enough to buy into the sporting metaphor—it was helpful during the rapid recovery from the second operation. But it didn't prepare me for chemo. Being a fat boy did that, a fat boy who had to learn to take it to survive—to face the bully and take it until he was strong enough to give it back.

Conventional wisdom in Queens when I was growing up in the fifties was that bullies would always back down if you stood up to them. This was simply not true. Most bullies had their own pride and constituencies to satisfy and they wouldn't have picked on you in the first place if they weren't sure they could beat you up. But it was a necessary lie that parents and older siblings had to tell us if we were ever to lose our fears. The important lesson was not about beating the bully, but about finding out that the beating he gave you was bearable, that he couldn't kill you. Simply by standing up to him and surviving you won a small victory that would give you the courage to keep challenging, to keep standing up, until he left you alone.

Chemo was like that, the bully you might outlast.

I learned to stand up to chemo when I was twelve, back in junior high school, Stephen A. Halsey, No. 157, in Rego Park, Queens. Oh, there were bullies in those days, Ronald and

Willie and Crazy Jay, who hung from the chain-link fence with one hand, throwing punches and snarling. We were lucky; no one fought with anything but fists and feet. I can only imagine what it means to stand up to a bully these days in city schools where a bully might shoot you, or at least slash you with a box-cutter. The chance to learn to fight back without dying is yet another loss in this time of the betrayal of children.

The schoolyard bully is never hard to spot; he's not necessarily bigger than the other kids, but he's always more physical, rolling his shoulders, moving his hands, getting up just a little too close. "You talkin' to me?" he says, before you have cleared your throat. That usually shuts you up.

At Halsey, I belonged to a group targeted by bullies. The members of the Special Progress class had been selected primarily by their above-average IQ scores (supposedly you had to be over 120), a fact we flaunted like a varsity letter. Not only were we smarter, but also we were too cool for this school; we would leave for high school after completing the three-year curriculum in two years. We were easy to resent. We traveled from class to class as a group and we could be individually identified by heavy brown-leather briefcases filled with books. The other kids made a sport of trying to kick them out of the hands of SP boys. They called our briefcases "fag bags."

"Fag" was the killer word in my neighborhood. In those days it had far less of a specifically homosexual connotation than one of "sissy," or worse, "girl." In the fifties, as we believed then, women had no real futures. They might become teachers or even writers, but they would never get to fly planes, build bridges, kill bad guys—real man's work. And this wasn't just schoolyard talk. One of the books in my bag, *The New You and Heredity,* had a chart that measured a man's masculinity by his line of work. The top of the masculinity chart drummed with test pilots, engineers, explorers. On the bottom, clearly my future neighborhood, were clergymen, teachers, and writers.

Bookish boys believe what they read and that chart burned into my brain like a diagram left too long on a computer screen. It was superimposed on everything that life scrolled up.

I was a particular target of the bullies because I was a compulsive smart-aleck who was also too fat to run away. (My weight has always been considerably higher than my IQ.) While the school tended to isolate us from the general student population, it didn't protect us. The principal, Dr. Herbert V. Nussey, who also taught Latin to the SP class and ran the schoolwide softball tournament, apparently believed in survival of the fittest. He would allow a little roughhouse as long as his authority wasn't challenged. Boys will be boys. Our SP home-room teacher, Mrs. McDermott, made an effort to stop fights before we were hurt, but she couldn't be everywhere. The official school enforcers, the burly gym and shop teachers, would wait until the fight was nearly over, then peel the bullies off their victims and boot them down the street in a humorous, bullying way that did nothing to condemn the ritual—in fact, it probably reinforced it. The bullies loved the attention, the contact with bully teachers. We victims dusted ourselves off and slunk home.

I hated getting beaten up. I hated having friends feel sorry for me, hated feeling my scabs harden while I listened to the conventional wisdom about standing up to bullies. But it seemed preferable to shutting up or making peace with the bullies. One of my SP classmates, Freddy, was famous for cozying up to "the hoods," as we called them—even holding their jackets while they beat us up. He went on to become a famous TV mogul.

At twelve and thirteen in my Halsey days, my major role model (I have yet to find a better one) was the Lone Ranger.

He protected people from bullies without ever being a bully himself. On Tuesday nights in the summertime, my father and I went to the cowboy movies—mostly grade-B black-and-white flicks. I think we liked being together more than we liked the films. It was our ballgame. Dad and I would have a soda afterward and discuss the superiority of Lash LaRue and the Durango Kid to the singing cowboys, Gene Autry and Roy Rogers, who rode the range with his wife.

The death of the Western movie was the death of a certain kind of masculine value system. Sex and violence were carefully separated. The hero might get the girl at the end, but that was romance, and nothing would happen between them until the credits had rolled. Usually he picked the nice girl over the saloon singer, but sometimes, especially if he had a bit of rough history himself, he went off with the whore with a heart of gold. By the sixties, when the Western hero had been replaced by James Bond, the line between fucking and fighting was gone. The hero rolled off the female vessel and returned fire at the terrorists coming through the window, who were often pals of the woman he had just pounded to orgasm. (Conveniently, she sometimes got killed in the crossfire.) And a little later, having just taken one in the arm, or slugged his way out of a jam, without much change of technique he'd go right into a clinch with a babe, still sweating, still squeezing them off one round at a time.

When I'd go to Westerns with my friends we'd discuss, on the way home, the perceived message: stand up to bullies or forever live in cowardice and shame. More than once, the morality play we had just seen became a rehearsal for reality. Tough kids from other neighborhoods would spot us even without our fag bags and cuff us around, snatch our hats. Paul and Jimmy and Mark and I, surrounded by a half-dozen teenagers wearing black leather and smoking Camels, would freeze, then struggle, and eventually take our lumps. Like men. No begging, no whimpering. It was brief and rarely brutal. Afterward, finding ourselves alive, we would swagger home revising the sad scuffle into the Gunfight at the O.K. Corral. We had survived without dishonor!

I was almost really hurt only once. Caught in a distant neighborhood at twilight on my bike, I was set upon by kids who chased me down a block. One of them threw a stick through the front wheel and I was thrown over the handle-bars, hands out. Nothing broken, but everything sprained. My ten jammed fingers looked like blue sausages for a week. Recovery brought the Nietzschean revelation—what doesn't kill you makes you stronger.

My regular bully was Willie, who had marked me in ele-mentary school, and followed me to Halsey. At P.S. 139, the grade school, teachers were alert to predatory kids, and be-cause I lived near school I could waddle away while Willie was being detained for questioning. Once home, I'd bury my shame with peanut butter sandwiches, Hydrox cookies, Her-shey bars, and wash down the lumps in my throat with a glass of chocolate milk.

But in the more Darwinian atmosphere at Halsey, where Willie was joined by other fag-bag kickers, I didn't stand a chance. At least once a week, he found me and roughed me up. Nothing much to see—a bruise, a little blood, a pocket half-torn off a shirt—but plenty to stew about. Willie was probably just a pathetic dork who had found a scapegoat for his unhappiness. But at the time, he was Grendel, and I was at the bottom of the masculinity chart.

I took it. I didn't get beaten up every day, in fact not even most days, but the fear of the beating was always there, as well as the humiliation of being so vulnerable to the fear. And to the name-calling—fag, fatso, lardass, Lippo the Hippo— that reduced me from whatever dream I had of myself to just being an object.

And then one day . . .

It was really no different from any other. The SP class was coming out of school at three o'clock with our usual mixed feelings. School was over, which was supposed to be a liberation, but school was where most of us found a comfortable arena and a sanctuary from the less-forgiving world of the street. Outside Halsey, the hoods capered around us, kicking at bags, calling us names. Willie found me and said something typically stupid. Typically, my smart-aleck reply made the other hoods laugh and infuriated Willie, who kicked my bag out of my hand. I stood and sneered at him.

And then—was it because Rose and Barbara were watching, because my hand really hurt this time, because something else was going on in my life?—I snapped. Suddenly, Willie became *my* target and object, the scapegoat for my inadequacies.

I hurled myself at Willie, just launched all that blubber like a rocket of rage. Surprisingly, we both went down. Incredibly, I was on top.

Had I known the protocols of the after-school fight, I would have sat on his stomach and tried to slap his head until he cried "Uncle." And he would have probably thrown me off and beaten me up once again. But I didn't know the rules, so I jammed my fat knees down into his lungs and grabbed fistfuls of his greasy hair and began to bash his brains out. Literally. I bounced his skull on the cold gray sidewalk as if it were a beachball. It was wonderful.

Mrs. McDermott screaming, "Robert! You'll hurt him!" sounded faint because I was roaring, "I'm gonna kill you!" and my friends were cheering and Willie was bawling and Crazy Jay dropped off the fence to clap. Then a shop teacher peeled me off and laughed as he put a steel-tipped toe in my rear and the principal grabbed me. It was years before I realized he was trying not to smile.

I suppose there are larger implications in all this about good and evil, war and peace, men and women, and overeating. But I'm sure only of this: I've been beaten up in many different ways since then, but I've never since thought of myself as a victim.

And Willie never bothered me again. (Nobody at Halsey ever did.) But he still lives in a little room in my head, which I visit whenever I need to remember who I want to be, what I need to be.

I would let Willie out of the little room whenever I went for chemo.

4

ON FRIDAY, September 1, we drove into the city to begin the two-year protocol of chemotherapy. Every Friday for six weeks I would get an intravenous injection, then every other week until the following September, then every three weeks for a year. There was a sense of adventure about it. Margie was up for the game and, at first, so was I.

The great moments of one's medical history usually belong to someone else—the brilliant diagnostician thrilled to discover your disease, the D'Artagnan of surgeons basking in the adoration of residents and nurses after a daring cut, the auditor discovering that an attending physician had put enough of his head into your room to justify his billing you for a visit. The tough moments are all yours.

The great Chemo Adventure began, as do so many adventures in New York City, with parking. The nearest lot to Memorial at the time, the one that chemo patients who might want to get home fast were advised to use, was directly across the street from the hospital. It was presided over by the kind of loud, crude, officious, stereotypical New Yorker you should only see in movies, a stumpy melon-head who looked and sounded as if he had missed the Mafia cut for private garbage jobs. Maybe the Godfather had gotten him this job by endowing a wing of the hospital.

He seemed to do most of his work from a folding metal-

and-mesh lawn chair, drinking coffee, yelling at a black assistant through a mouthful of doughnut. It's not as if we hadn't suffered such characters all our lives, but usually we could growl back, walk away, or be cool and think, hey, I can deal with this now; he's probably got worse problems.

Well, at the time the only people I considered to have worse problems were people in more advanced stages of cancer. And we would have to get into this parking lot, past this stumpy melon-headed jerk, every Friday morning for six weeks, then every other Friday morning, then every third Friday morning unless, of course, I died or he got cancer.

Do I sound angry? Probably even angrier than I felt at the time. But talking about it then helped me, and dredging up that anger all these years later is easy. The hospital has since put an office building on that parking lot, but the casual cruelty still exists (although there have been major improvements in some areas) and, of course, that feeling of vulnerability in the face of that cruelty still exists.

For someone like me, who rarely expressed extreme emotional feelings in those days, there was something enormously helpful in sounding off about doctors, nurses, aides, techs, parking attendants who seemed insensitive to the fragility of a patient. Suffering in silence is often necessary simply because few people want to hear your complaints, and, after a while, if you get the reputation of being a "krock," they'll find ways to ignore you, which can be deadly. Here was a guy we had to be nice to, even tip generously, because we were at his mercy. But to keep up our spirits, to keep that 'tude alive, there had to be a way of getting back at him, even if only privately.

Make a fist, but keep it in your pocket. I learned diplomatic restraint in that parking lot. Make a nasty comment, but don't let it pass your lips. I learned to keep my eye on the prize, not to be distracted from the goal of getting in and out of Memorial as quickly as possible.

As a white male of a fifties' sensibility, I took my entitlements for granted; with an Ivy League education, no discernible handicaps, and a willingness to shave and wear a tie, I assumed I would always get by. I'm Jewish, but that's less of a strike against me in New York than anywhere else but Tel Aviv. I believed devoutly in integration, and I believed in a level playing field for women. I felt I was about as far from being prejudiced as I could be.

But all that was theoretical. It took illness to make me feel powerless and to eventually offer some insight into what it might really mean to be black, a female, gay, and have to grovel, flirt, cakewalk, conceal. Much later, feeling entitled again, I could try to integrate these new insights into my writings and my actions. This was a positive side effect, a useful souvenir from Malady.

But in the fall of 1978, traveling in-country, I used those insights in a cruder way—to give myself permission to get off racially, sexually, ethnically on people I thought were oppressing me. Making jokes was part of a venting system. If you have no other way of striking back, at least you can silently call a jerk a Mafia melon-head. Pathetic, to be sure, but it helped me.

Dealing with that border guard was also good preparation for one Malady travel skill that I am still refining, the ability to cultivate "good relationships" (call it finesse, call it Tomming) with all those gatekeepers who do not seem involved in the medical implications of their jobs. They might as well be guarding the door of a bank, a welfare office, corporate headquarters. They assume that you have come to do wrong, cheat on food stamps, kidnap the boss, at the least annoy them while they are having a second breakfast.

It's bad enough when such people are giving you a hard time at the motor vehicle bureau. At the illness bureau you feel as though they are threatening your life, which they may be. You have to go into survival mode, and you have to do it

in your own fashion. Don't be shy about intimidating or ca-
joling. I'm not good at either. I can't even scare babies. When
I try to be nice and chatty, I come off seeming insincere,
which I am. People often brought gifts, even to doctors, but
certainly to the gatekeepers—flowers to receptionists, candy
to nurses, coffee and doughnuts to parking-lot guardians.

Margie felt very strongly about such bribes: "Millions for
defense, not one cent for tribute!" And I agreed with her. In-
tegrity! Dignity! However, as we became more sophisticated
in our travels, we saw how Malady often demanded new definitions of what was considered appropriate behavior. After
all, in everyday life one rarely cracks the savings account for
the privilege of stripping naked for strangers. The trick, as always, is to be yourself and to survive.

In general, Margie, who was not particularly patient, was
far more patient through my chemo adventure than I was. At
the time, I thought it might be a gender characteristic: Weren't
women better than men at accommodating, at waiting things
out? We were on the cresting wave of the women's movement
then, and there was much talk of sex role differences. Eventually, our travels in Malady offered up a different answer. Her
patience through my illness—and my patience through hers—
had nothing to do with gender and everything to do with assuming the role of caregiver. Patients may allow themselves a
certain selfishness, especially when they sense it is tolerated,
just like a pro athlete, sitcom star, or child. But the caregiver
must be a grown-up, steady and responsible. In many ways it
is the tougher job, and the smart patient never willfully com-
plicates it.

As our Malady partnership took shape, we tended to act
in ways comfortable to our personalities. Outgoing Margie
liked to talk with other people. I closed up into myself, a
variation of Greg's thousand-yard stare. She said she got
medical information as well as story ideas, but I knew that

chattering was one way she dispelled anxiety. And as much as I might say I was conserving energy for the ordeal, we both understood that I was simply shutting down systems to avoid anxiety. Were there better ways for us to respond? Maybe. But these worked for us.

By the time we reached Memorial, I was usually a punctured, crumpled beachball. On my best days I was simply there, waiting for the Baby Don to yell at his assistant through his doughnut, slurp his coffee, then grandly wave us through, for which we paid in advance with something extra for him. It all probably transpired in ten minutes, but for me it seemed forever.

Then we went into the hospital and took a number, as in a bakery. No matter when we arrived there were always many people ahead of us, often in family clumps. The patient would usually be the father or mother, in their sixties or seventies, with one or two middle-aged daughters, the son or son-in-law who drove them in from the suburbs, perhaps a grandchild or two. Invariably, someone would be clutching a large manila envelope of X-rays. When I wasn't tucked into my own protective box, I would watch them act out their accustomed roles in the family. The clown made jokes, the weepy one turned away to dab her eyes. The strong daughter summoned nurses and doctors, ordered a sibling to get food, sternly told Dad that Mom would be all right, she had found her the best doctor in the house.

There were also similar groups from foreign countries, a clutch of rich Italians or Argentines, well-dressed and grim. There were always couples in fashion denial—tennis outfits in summer, après-ski in winter—and occasional familiar faces, even stars. More than once I saw the lawyer Roy Cohn float ghostlike through the waiting room. This flashed back many years later when Cohn was a character dying in the play *Angels in America*. There would be recognizable actor faces, although we couldn't always recall the names, and once I spotted a very large young man I couldn't quite place.

Toward the end of chemo I found out he was a New York Giants linebacker named Dan Lloyd, who had lymphoma. In an amazing turn, when I went into television in 1982, he would be the subject of my first on-air story. He beat chemo, but he was cut from the team—the Giants apparently thought his bones would be too brittle to take the pounding. Dan was disappointed because beating chemo, recovering, wasn't enough. As it was to all of us, victory was a return to ordinary life, and his ordinary life was knocking down quarterbacks in the NFL.

There was also a disproportionate number of gay couples. There were middle-aged men sitting close, the so-called "clones" with their matching biceps and mustaches, and a few leather boys. Long before I had any idea of AIDS, my chemo host, Tom Reynolds, mentioned that something mysterious was going around. He said he didn't want to be in New York when it really hit.

IF I WAS UP for it, I could get involved figuring the order in which to check off the pre-chemo chores, the finger-stick to be sure my blood count was high enough to handle the heavy juice, perhaps even a full blood test, a chest X-ray to see if the cancer had reached my lungs, the weigh-in and the blood pressure exam. The game of it was to reckon—by the length of the lines and the look of the patients—if there was time to run downstairs for a chest X-ray before the finger-stick. I soon learned that my lungs were unusually wide and long, good for breathing but awkward for placement in the standard X-ray machines. I needed a special machine. Sometimes that meant a longer wait but sometimes I would be taken immediately because that machine happened to be free. The women who ran the X-ray counter and handed out little brass tokens for the lockers were generally suspicious of my special request, but I found that if I apologetically told them that I needed "the wide-bodied machine for fat guys" they immediately smiled at me, told me I wasn't fat, and were helpful. At first, I resented having to soap them up just to be treated with ordinary courtesy. But eventually I got pleasure out of the exchanges. I felt that I was not entirely at their mercy, that I was taking charge of the situation. I could even make believe that I was not groveling so much as learning a language. I was being cool.

The upbeat, noncommittal friendliness of the X-ray technicians made a difference. It was comforting. Because they checked the X-rays before releasing the patient, there was always the sense that they knew if the picture showed bad news. They were only checking to see that the picture had come out clearly, but I always studied their faces for a grimace, watched to see if they averted their eyes, a sure sign they had spotted a suspicious shadow. But they always smiled cheerfully.

The outpatient blood-gatherers were a less cheerful lot, and I don't know if it was occupational or cultural. Often they were Asian men and women impatient when the blood didn't flow quickly enough out of my veins and into their tubes. "You haven't been drinking enough liquids," they would accuse, unless, of course, there was too much blood too quickly, in which case they accused me of having gobbled aspirin the night before. In the spirit of Bobby Finesse, I would usually confess to any accusation and swear never to do it again, especially while they were still jabbing away. This is not something I would recommend anywhere else in Malady—giving false information can be very dangerous—but these people were not making decisions; they were just stabbing me. While the finger-sticks always hurt—why were they often more painful than a jab in the elbow vein?—it was the intravenous needlework that still stitches the Memorial samplers of my mind.

The blood-workers tended to be stylists. There were the "tailors," slow and careful, sliding in their needles right under the skin. When they hit blood immediately, they were the best, but they rarely hit blood immediately and when nothing came out they would begin manipulating the needle inside the vein, scratching around, which was almost always a painful waste of time.

Then there were the "top sticks," usually younger men, often Hispanic, who would plunge the needle straight down from a foot away. It was scary. I never got used to it because I rarely saw the same guy twice in a row, but on average they were the best. It was amazing how often they struck a gusher.

Always the worst were the "jabbers," usually former nurse's aides up from the ranks, who took short, quick, almost tentative hits at veins and missed as often as they hit. They were the ones who would accuse me of having slippery veins, for which I would usually apologize.

I rated outpatient blood-gatherers with ouches—one to four—and came to know the good ones and the bad ones. Not that there were choices. I'd start smiling if one of the good ones was on duty, trying to lure her over with positive magnetic energy. I'd chat up the bad ones, try to relax them, especially in the second year when the big veins in my elbows, buffeted by chemo and jabs, began to scar up, and it became necessary to go to the veins in my hands, which are smaller and more difficult to hit. Hand hits are also more painful.

I still make a practice of chatting up the blood-gatherers, asking them how they feel, apologizing for making them work the little hand veins, trying to give them the sense that I understand—which I do—how tense and demanding their jobs are. I make it clear that I'm an old hand, pun intended, and I won't go through the roof if they hurt me a little. I like to think this calms them down, and I know for sure it calms me down; I'm also pretty sure that over the years, it has reduced the ouches.

Chatting up the outpatient aides who weighed me and took my blood pressure was risky. They tended to be very sensitive about their inferior position and were quick to flash attitude if they thought they were being patronized. On the other hand, if you weren't sociable, if you were grumpy, they took it personally. I also learned never to interrupt if they were in the middle of one of their interminable discussions with a fellow aide about lunch or the subways or those uppity nurses who thought their shit was frozen yogurt.

On days when things were moving smoothly, dealing with these natives of Malady could be diverting, could actually make you forget about the reason you were there. On bad days, you felt like jumping out of your skin. It's another good reason to have someone steady by your side.

Based on the count of red and white blood cells and platelets from the finger-stick test, the doctors made the decision as to whether or not you would actually get chemo that day. A low count could mean infections, anemia, poor clotting, and might make it necessary to postpone chemo until you were in better shape to take the assault. Except for a little cancer, I was remarkably healthy. In two years, I remember only one time that my count was too low for chemo.

This was the point at which I would be seen by a doctor, usually either the merry Davor Vugrin or Tom Reynolds, whose importance in keeping me going cannot be overstated. Tom was sometimes flighty, and could make outrageous pronouncements, but he was also so honest and grounding that I trusted him to always tell the truth.

Tom was interested in art, in our writings, and thus our

brief pre-chemo exams—rarely lasting more than five or ten minutes—would be flecked with friendly cocktail-party chatter that made an enormous difference in my mood. Tom's enthusiasm for getting on with procedures and then back to everyday life, his implicit assurance that all this was a necessary, but not defining, aspect of my existence swept me along for most of the first year. Of course, that enthusiasm could become frightening too.

One Friday in November of that first year, while I was going through the bakery line, Margie went downtown to the Strang Clinic for a general cancer screening. While she was gone, a Memorial radiologist had spotted a suspicious mass on the X-ray of my lungs. There was a sudden flurry. With urgency in her voice, a nurse called me into an examining room out of turn. I was swarmed by Tom, Davor, and several doctors I had never seen before. I did not fully understand what they were talking about, but Tom was clearly opting to "crack his chest right away" and Davor was muttering into his beard. I was sent for another X-ray, and experts further up the med chain were alerted.

The doctors went off to confer over lunch and left me alone for an hour in the vast outpatient waiting room, awash with a panic that felt like waves of alternating hot and cold water surging through my body. It took awhile to get my brain under control, to think it through. If there was a tumor in my lungs, there could also be tumors in my liver and brain.

At the very least, it would mean an operation, then more and harsher chemo, like the cisplatin we'd all been so happy was invented, the stuff that had hooked Sergeant Alec to a dialysis machine.

At worst, it could be the beginning of an extended, painful slide to death. I tried to focus on what I needed to do to get my life in order—will, parents, wife, kids, current projects wrapped up. Since the initial diagnosis, I had kept all financial records up to the minute. I could afford to think about an early alternative to a long, hard dying.

Because the word "suicide" seemed too harsh, I thought in terms of "checking out." I imagined checking out with a skyscraper jump, a bullet to the roof of my mouth, an overdose of barbiturates, even diving in front of a subway train. But these all seemed messy, leaving problems for other people. Worse, all had margins of error that could leave me in really bad shape, a vegetable with cancer.

I remembered one summer afternoon, as a teenager, when I dove beneath the raft in the middle of the lake and couldn't find my way out from under. Panicky, thrashing, I kept bumping up against the bottom of the raft as the cold water sapped my strength. A moment came when I thought I was going to die and with it came a wonderful sense of numb peace. And then, of course, I popped to the surface, breaking through to a glorious gasp of delicious air I can still taste today.

Sitting alone in the waiting room, I imagined swimming out to sea, perhaps into the Caribbean, farther and farther, beyond the sounds of the beach and the flashes of holiday sails until the waves would gather me under forever. No fuss, no mess. I felt peaceful and liberated. I had found a clean way to go. It got me through the hour.

This, of course, is not the only way to get through those dreadful times when you are helplessly anticipating bad news. Some people can lose themselves in a book, movie, video game, a conversation, intense exercise if you are able to be that physical. Later, when I became a regular yoga student, I found that deep breathing helped enormously. By concentrating on the breaths, imagining a white silk scarf moving in and out of my body as I silently counted out four-second intervals of breathing in, holding it, then breathing out, I could blot out all other thoughts for enough time to reduce my terror.

But that particular terror time, Margie remembered coming back from Strang to find me pale and catatonic. The terror had imprisoned me. Eventually, the doctors came back from lunch chuckling at an eager young resident anxious to find something his elders had missed. He had misinterpreted something they called an "artifact," a shadow of a bone. Everything was fine. It wasn't time to check out after all.

So now I could go on to the chemo room.

Sitting in one of the molded plastic chairs that lined the wall across from the chemo room, I hoped for a good nurse. Most of the chemo nurses were Sheilas—she had been one—cheerful, tough, steady. But there were "jabbers" here, too. By this time, however, much of the anticipatory fear and loathing of the day was over for me. I was almost done. Once I got the chemo I could go home, not think about this for another week or two (early in the second year, the three-week interval felt like a vacation).

Once inside the room, on a chair (the beds and recliners were reserved for people who had chemo drips that lasted for hours), my mood brightened. A nurse approached with my bag of drugs and I'd start pumping my fist to get the veins swelling.

Every so often I'd draw a clumsy nurse who told me that I was the only person who had ever given her "trouble." After two or three jabs, and then long, digging attempts to get in, I'd tell her to quit and get me a supervisor. They might glare, but they always did, and they seemed relieved.

Most of the time, it went fine. I got what was called a "push." The actual infusion of drugs and the saline solution that adulterated them enough to keep them from burning out my veins lasted no more than twenty minutes. The worst that could happen, and it occasionally did, was that chemo would leak out of a vein into the surrounding tissue, where it burned its way up to the skin. Swollen hands and green-black bruises were common. A severe injury was possible. It was the main reason to want a competent nurse.

The protocol that Davor Vugrin had finally chosen was the so-called mini-VAB, the lowest dosage of chemo, a cocktail of vinblastine, actinomycin D, and bleomycin, plus chlorambucil taken orally at home. Years later, Tom Reynolds would tell me that he had argued for a higher dosage because my alpha protein markers, signals of disease, had not come down quickly after the operations. Davor had agonized over his decision for a year or more, wondering if he had given me enough chemo. I assured him it felt like plenty.

You can actually feel chemo drugs enter your bloodstream. There is a chilly prickle as the first chemo bubble slides out of a silver needle into your vein, a subtle sensation of vibration, almost a buzzing in the vein, then a rising heat that eventually becomes a distinct burning. I could imagine flames on water, an oil fire on Lake Erie. As the chemo traveled farther from the site of the push, I would lose track of it.

Once the needle came out, I would be given a white vomit bag for the trip home. The worst was over. Now it was just a matter of being sick for a day or two.

Chemo is a cumulative experience, physically as well as emotionally. The relentlessness of it wears you down and the accumulation of toxic wastes in your body makes you progressively sicker after each treatment. And then there is the Pavlovian conditioning to anticipating being sick. At the start of treatment, I wouldn't throw up until five or six hours after the push. That was plenty of time to drive back to suburban New Jersey, have some food, get comfortable in bed with the radio on and water nearby, and prepare for three or four hours of vomiting and retching, usually at fifteen-minute intervals, before I collapsed into sleep. In the beginning, I might even reappear in the early evening, tired and sore, to watch TV.

I usually felt lousy the next day, hung over, my throat raw, stomach upset. Neal Conan said to think of it as a date with a bad piece of shellfish. Such smart, useful encouragement was more important than even Conan, war correspondent, prizewinner, could ever know.

Toward the end of the two years, I became nauseated on the drive in to Memorial—the Baby Don knew us well by this time and had mellowed into a low-level rudeness—and I was retching myself into unconsciousness for the rest of the night.

For ten years afterward, I'd get queasy going back for checkups. My stomach would flip just driving near that neighborhood. As I write this eighteen years after that first chemo shot, I take deep breaths, trying to fight off lightheadedness, tingling in my arms, a distant rumble in my bowels.

ORDINARY LIFE went on along with chemo. Or, more accurately, chemo became part of ordinary life. We went to the opera, we went bowling, we went to see the leaves turn in the Berkshires and to see the kids in school plays.

My hair began to fall out, first while I brushed it, then under the shower spray. People were wearing ice packs on their heads during chemo to slow the loss, but I never felt that concerned about my crowning glory. About half my hair fell out—actually it thinned out—and I looked merely male-pattern baldish. That winter, during a book-signing at a library convention, a woman came by and made some lame joke about my having less hair in person than in my book-jacket photo. I found that hilarious and life-affirming. Not only did she never suspect I had cancer, but she was also clumsily trying to pick me up, exposed scalp and all. The kid was coming back.

I never considered myself in grave danger, and I never was. As time goes on and I become more sophisticated about cancer, the word alone has little resonance. What kind of cancer are we talking about, and at what stage?

Which is not to say I didn't use cancer to give myself permission to act like a jerk. In an incident for which I still feel embarrassed, soon after I began chemo I had lunch with a successful television writer deeply involved in social causes, and I asked him how he could take such progressive political stances and still write such violent low-level crap. He was knocked back but recovered to mumble something about working from within the system. The opportunity to apologize has never presented itself. Who am I to be so righteous? But what could I say now? That the mini-VAB was talking, not me? You sure?

I finished my thriller and my editor wrote a letter telling me how much he hated it and why he wouldn't publish it. I put the manuscript in a bottom drawer, where it still is. What can I say? The mini-VAB wrote the final draft?

Margie finished her novel, and her editor loved it. So did I. In 1980, Doubleday published *Hot Type,* a smart, woman's-cye view of what she called "The Paper." Margie had worked at the *New York Times,* where we met, at a time when there were few women on staff, and none of the present commitment to hiring more women or minority reporters and editors.

The media critic of the *Los Angeles Times* reviewed *Hot Type* unfavorably on the front page of his paper's Sunday book review in a curiously male and patronizing way that made reference to his own wife, contentedly reading at his side. I wondered if the Cancer Man would take the assignment, and give me a discount as a fellow patient.

Drugs such as Compazine and nabilone, then given in various forms, such as pills, injections, or suppositories, to combat nausea never really worked for me, so I decided to inhale. Several very good friends sent or brought me bags of marijuana. But pot never did much for me either, although many people have been helped enormously. The continued prohibitions against medical use seem immoral.

I once had what seemed like a wonderful drug-induced hallucination. Finger-stuck and X-rayed, I went out on the street one day to smoke a joint before my chemo push. Suddenly, as Margie and I strolled near the hospital, a woman we knew, the wife of a colleague, floated toward us, actually floated above the sidewalk, I thought. Her voice wrapped around us like stereo: "He did it with a stewardess, that fuck, and now I'm going to take him for every cent he has. I'm on my way to see my lawyer, Roy Cohn."

Then she floated on. I was thrilled at the apparition. The pot was finally working. I was so relaxed that I had an easy chemo infusion, laughed at the jabs. But I still vomited all night. I gave up using marijuana soon after that. Years later, I told my colleague the story of my reefer madness. He laughed bitterly. It had really happened, he said. He was still paying off Cohn's legal fees.

THAT CANCEROUS summer, when I was taking sitz baths and antibiotics prescribed by local doctors, I was also writing press releases at the South Bronx election campaign headquarters of Ramon Jimenez, who was running for the state senate. I admired Ramon, a young lawyer whom I had met during a brief column-writing stint for the *New York Post* the year before. I also liked the Puerto Ricans who flowed through his office and his life. Their macho style seemed very ornate, almost self-conscious in the late seventies, when men were having to deal with a new wave of feminism that demanded not only equality but also a dialing-down of traditional masculinity.

So I had mixed feelings about these swaggering Latins in Ramon's office. My newly found feminine side was repelled:

Weren't they the enemy, the lip-smacking sexists on the street who touched bouncing braless women?

But my retrograde masculine side enjoyed their cockiness. Ramon himself, a graduate of Harvard Law, was not ostentatiously macho, but the gypsy cab drivers and hospital workers who flocked to his campaign could only be described as ballsy, and I felt that way myself in their presence.

But the friend of Ramon who most engaged my memory was Carmen, a single mother of three who had put herself through college by cheating on welfare and taking a taste of anything that passed. She had even enthusiastically looted a neighborhood supermarket during the 1977 New York City blackout. She was a very tough survivor. She was proud, assertive, involved in community protests and fiercely attentive to her children. I didn't understand everything she did, but I sensed she was prepared to do anything necessary to go the distance, one day at a time.

The cocky guys and their Latin dance macho faded out, but Carmen grew sharper as the chemo accumulated in my body and my nausea and vomiting got worse. I was always looking for little lessons, metaphors, new ways to get myself up to keep pushing on. Just believing that I needed the chemo to kill off all the stray little cancer cells floating in my body wasn't enough. Maybe they were all dead already; or maybe they were successfully hiding in ambush, waiting for my immune system to drop its guard again.

I had to think this was some kind of test, that I had to go the distance to prove myself worthy. To stop would be to hit myself with a rifle butt to avoid the twenty-mile hike. And yet, the best example I had seen of someone going the distance was a welfare mom in the South Bronx. Carmen was the essence of what I came to believe was true manhood. Hanging tough. (She still is, working and living in the Bronx, as is Ramon, a respected college professor and labor lawyer.)

With a lot of time to think in those days, lying in darkened rooms, sipping water, recovering from four or five hours of throwing up, I often thought about sex and manhood, both specifically—I was still too chopped up to have sex, but what would it be like once I did?—and abstractly.

Had I—had my generation—learned the rules of manhood? Had we been properly tested and certified? Maybe the reason my generation was skipped over from ultimate elective power—the presidency went from World War II Warrior George Bush to Boomer Bill Clinton—was because we hadn't been tested. We'd missed all the potholes and speed bumps. The great traumas were all vicarious for us. Born at the end of the Depression, too young to fight in World War II or Korea, too old for Vietnam, we also missed the full kicks of drugs, sex, and rock 'n' roll. Maybe our lack of confidence showed. Would chemo be my war?

Still a bookish boy, I began reading about cancer, although I never became a student of the disease. There were three books I read during those chemo years that were important to me, all by professional writers who approached their illnesses in idiosyncratic ways. Although I found each book foreign to my own experience and sometimes off-putting, each of them helped me find my own way.

I was well into chemo when Norman Cousins's *Anatomy of an Illness as Perceived by the Patient* arrived to great acclaim. The book was a description of his recovery from a serious disease of the connective tissues fifteen years earlier, and his larger thoughts on medicine and the role of the patient. The book was thoughtful and fresh, and hopeful; it urged patients to take at least partial responsibility for their own healing, not to turn over control of their lives to the medical biz.

How I hated that book at first, and without good reason. What right did Cousins have to write a best-seller when I was the only truly sick writer in the world? I skimmed the book in a jealous fury, and allowed myself to be guided by reviewers

and commentators who also missed his major points and ap-
plauded the "laughter as the best medicine" angle; to raise
his spirits and endorphins, Cousins had screened film come-
dies and read humor books (there were also massive intravenous doses of self-prescribed Vitamin C). He opined that
those who survived serious illness tended to have a "robust
will to live," along with faith in their doctors. He wrote:
"Cancer, in particular, has been connected to intensive states
of grief or anger or fear. It makes little sense to suppose that
emotions exact only penalties and exact no benefits."

No wonder the medical establishment was showering him
with fellowships and teaching gigs, I raged. He gives doctors
the ultimate escape hatch—the patient's faith or will to live
wasn't strong enough. It all fit in with "blaming the victim,"
I thought.

But the thesis of Cousins's book was much more than
laughing ("jogging for the innards," he called it) and wishing
to get well. In a nonthreatening way, without trash talk,
anger, or tumor humor, he carefully and persuasively made
his case for the doctor-patient partnership being at the core
of healing. As I came back to the book again and again over
the years, I realized how wise it was—and more and more
unsettling. In a time of managed care, of prescribed-to-the-
minute limits on medical "face time," that core may now be
hollow.

Consider this, from Cousins: "Time is the one thing that
patients need most from their doctors—time to be heard,
time to have things explained, time to be reassured, time to
be introduced by the doctor personally to specialists or other
attendants whose very existence seems to reflect something
new and threatening."

As I dip back into Cousins's book, I feel even more
strongly that the best basic partnership is between the patient
and the designated caregiver—be it parent, spouse, child,

trusted friend, paid sidekick—who can act as extra ears and eyes, as gopher, cheerleader, advisor. The relationship between a doctor and a patient can never be a relationship between equals, the prerequisite for partnership. The doctor must ration time, must practice triage, must weigh possible result against potential cost. The patient—quite properly worrying about only one patient—wants all the attention and resources that will give him a chance at recovery. The doctor and the patient are quite often not on the same page; managed care is the handiest current villain, but the demands of a needy patient have always strained the medical system. Even something as low-tech as the simple "history," the pen-and-paper interview of a patient, has been routinely compressed into a quickie "What seems to be the problem?" The full-scale interview, including the patient's family medical history and everyday habits, is becoming rarer, even though experts believe that as many clues emerge from that face-to-face encounter as from a battery of high-tech tests. There's no time for the long interview because there is no short-term profit in it. And forget about the housecall, which so often gave the bright doctor a chance to play detective and find diagnostic clues in the refrigerator, the cat hairs, the peeling paint. The caregiver often becomes the critical factor in making the truncated doctor-patient meeting work, preparing questions in order of importance, making sure they are delivered forcefully (perhaps in advance of the visit by fax, E-mail, voice mail) and that they are answered. Staunch sidekicks are more likely than patients to hang tough as a doctor sighs and looks at his watch.

Susan Sontag's *Illness as Metaphor* was another book to which I had a bad early reaction. That one I threw across the room (highly aberrational—my father, a book collector, taught my sister and me to revere books as the sacred relics of civilization and as the magic carpets that would take us to places better than wherever we were). I think I reacted so viscerally to Sontag's book because in almost a hundred pages she never mentioned, much less engaged, what I considered the central fact of her book's existence, and the only reason to have written it—she was recovering from breast cancer. Why hide that, shoving cancer further into the closet?

I was wrong again. At least I learned never to trust a cancer reaction. Sontag dealt with her own cancer in her own cool, academic way. Eventually I would recognize the book as a classic, albeit an abstract, intellectual one, as Cousins's had been warm and immediately practical. Sontag's avowed purpose was to liberate us from the terrifying metaphors of illness so that we could regard illness realistically. By treating cancer as "an evil, invincible predator, not just a disease," she wrote, patients become "demoralized." People are reported to have died just from hearing their diagnosis—another anecdote for Cousins and the mind-over-metastasis crowd. I keep this in mind as I call disease "The Beast." Metaphors are okay as long as they don't overwhelm you.

The third book was *A Private Battle* by Cornelius Ryan and Kathryn Morgan Ryan, which is still the best book I've read about the terrible stress that a disease imposes on a family and its friends: ". . . the doctor's findings had already begun to make a difference," wrote Kathryn. "Cancer had separated us, a barrier, invisible but everlasting, had come between us."

Cornelius Ryan, a dashing former war correspondent, was the best-selling author of *The Longest Day* and *A Bridge Too Far,* the book he was working on in August 1970, when Dr. Whitmore, "the Cary Grant of medicine," as he described him in *A Private Battle,* diagnosed his prostate cancer. I was disturbed to read that Whitmore, a leading character in the book, might have made an error in judging the extent of the disease. He advised a watch-and-wait approach; but Ryan insisted on lymphangiography, that fascinating test that began with an incision into the foot. The dye that coursed through Ryan's body and was tracked by radiologists showed that the cancer ("like a demented mass murderer," wrote Kathryn) had metastasized. Whitmore would later insist he would have soon picked that up himself. Ryan died in Memorial in 1974. He was fifty-four.

In his sections of the book, Ryan had sharp and, unfortunately, still valid comments on the arrogance of doctors and their lack of communication with one another, much less with patients. He was well aware that the expertise and financial resources available for his personal medical research were out of the reach of most patients. This was a wealthy and well-connected man who went to Malady first-class, yet his wife still had to run screaming into the corridor to find someone to alleviate his pain.

There was such a strong narrative flow to the book that I wondered more than once if Kathryn could have written more of it than she let on. Cornelius's portions were supposedly edited from an immense file of medical reports, letters, notes he had secreted in a bottom drawer, and from twelve hours of tapes that neither she nor his secretary knew about until after his death. If so, illness had indeed separated them, since she had been deeply involved in every aspect of his personal and professional life until then.

She was a professional writer herself with an ego that had been squelched. Their biggest battle was over her request for a double byline to reflect her contribution to his acclaimed war histories. In the end, Kathryn wrote the most powerful of their books and gave Cornelius a byline.

I QUIT CHEMO on June 3, 1980, about a month earlier than scheduled, because suddenly I wanted to leave Malady, to return to ordinary life immediately. It was a totally personal decision; I had reached my limit. But after almost two years, it was not considered a risky move. If the juice hadn't killed all the little buggers by now, I figured, it probably never would.

Somewhere, hiding in a vena cava, lazing on the islets of Langerhans, might be one outlaw cell waiting for the toxic cloud to pass, for the day after Judgment to dawn so it could rise and multiply and start traveling and take me over. I would take that chance. I didn't want to vomit any more.

It was not a dramatic decision. I was scheduled for a regular chemo treatment on May 30, but Dr. Vugrin canceled, for the first time, and rescheduled for June 3. If he was getting that relaxed, I decided, so could I. He seemed to think it was okay. The last time I had felt so totally relieved was when I changed my college major to English from pre-med. I kept visiting Vugrin every few weeks. There were blood tests and chest X-rays and the careful finger crawl for swollen glands. And every time, he would write on my chart "NED." No evidence of disease.

It was a wonderful, ordinary summer. We swam every day, the kids went to a great camp for July, then we all spent a marvelous August in a house on a lake in the Berkshires. I read Proust, cooked Chinese food in a wok, finished a book that was published and a screenplay that was never produced. I even created a superhero.

Once I realized that I wouldn't have to become the Cancer Man, the dying mob executioner, I decided I would become Captain Cancer, a patient who got superhuman powers from his chemo treatments. This all came from a story I began telling Sam when he was pulling me out of soft chairs.

It was about a teenager who had gotten an experimental cancer drug that turned him fat and green and hairless. But it also gave him tremendous physical strength, the ability to see through walls and hear sounds a mile away. At first he was bewildered and scared by his powers, then thrilled, especially when his girlfriend helped him use them to bring some environmental villains to justice.

Sam liked the stories, but I loved them. I got chills making them up; I sometimes cried at my own storytelling, although that might have been the hormone swings.

Years later, I actually wrote a Young Adult novel called *The Chemo Kid,* which people tended not to understand; it was not realistic enough for the librarians who had gotten used to my grittier stories, and it had too many tasteless jokes for teachers who had never had cancer. So it didn't get into the hands of too many kids, who being kids would know they could laugh at the tumor humor.

Then again, the librarians and the teachers may have been right. I may have allowed the book to become one big location joke—you had to have been there to appreciate it, no thank you. The editor hated the ending, in which the Chemo Kid decided to keep on taking chemo even though he didn't need it any more, just so he could keep his superpowers. The editor didn't want to publish that ending because he thought it was a tacit approval of drug use. It was Sam, by now twenty-two and a writer, who came up with the solution. The Chemo Kid would be offered a drug that would return him to a normal appearance but cancel his superhuman powers.

So the Chemo Kid just said no.

BY THE END of that magical summer of 1980, I had decided that I was better for having had cancer, less likely to sweat the small stuff, bolder, harder to intimidate, more loving with friends and nastier with enemies.

I had less than eight months to wallow in all this self-improvement before Margie got her own diagnosis of cancer.

5

SUSANNAH ONCE described her feelings of mounting horror and helplessness as she watched me drive into a traffic accident. She was driving a half-block behind me as I made a tight right turn alongside a truck making a tighter right turn. The truck driver and I both miscalculated the room we had, or perhaps neither of us was willing to give ground. Metal skins rubbed against each other, the noise worse than the damage.

Susannah, trailing, saw it all very clearly, in slow motion. She was helpless to stop it, too far away to shout a warning. She could only hope it wouldn't happen, then that it wouldn't be so bad, then that she could be of use after it was over.

Meanwhile, I was totally involved in the action. Until it was over and she told me what she saw, I had only impressions of a scene that went by in an instant. I think of that scrape when people ask me about the difference between my first cancer and Margie's. During the early, anxious days of discovery and diagnosis, Margie's cancer was scarier for me than my own. I was scared for her, for me, for the kids, for our lives. There would be responsibility for me as a caregiver. The slow motion gave me more time for anxieties. Would I be adequate to the job? Would it become my life's work? Then I felt guilty for thinking about myself at such a time.

This is fairly standard, I later learned. It is probably impossible to avoid these anxieties; they may be a wasteful drain on your energy, but they are not off the wall. People do become consumed by caregiving. You should never feel guilty for thinking of yourself too. After all, if you burn out, get sick, lose heart, who will take care of the patient?

I've been close to several couples locked in what seemed to be destructive patient-caregiver relationships. In one, a retired doctor had given over his life to caring for his wife, who was suffering from advanced Alzheimer's disease. She could not be left alone because she might wander away or burn down the house. Although he could afford it, he refused to hire help, even the hourly "babysitting" that would allow him to get out of the house for a few hours at a time. He said he did not want his "privacy" intruded upon. Was it pride, guilt, obstinacy, shame? At this writing, his friends, who remember the wife's wit and charm, invite them to meals and parties and try to find ways to give him respite from her care, but they all fear that his nerves are fraying from the strain.

One fifty-year-old woman who lived in a one-room walk-up apartment could not afford outside care for her seventy-year-old husband, who had been disabled by a stroke. She refused to put him in a nursing home because she felt that those available to Medicaid patients were "hellholes." In her desperation, she sometimes tied him to a chair when she went out. Once she even took him to a doctor's appointment, left him in the waiting room, and fled the city for a week. Eventually, she did put him in a nursing home.

These are cautionary tales, but I'm not sure the lessons are clear-cut. As an acquaintance of the retired doctor, I could admire his devotion to his wife but not his refusal to get professional help. As a reporter writing about the other couple, I found it wrenching to watch her make the decision that left her free but nearly crazed with guilt.

Since most people are cared for at home, it is usually a family member who becomes a patient's closest, most critical

traveling companion in Malady. Since we have not yet figured out the proper care of all patients, it may be a little early
to stump for proper care of caregivers. So for starters, we
have to take care of ourselves, even if it means setting limits
on the demands of people we love. I know it sounds useless
to say, "Don't feel guilty for taking care of yourself," when I
can't always follow that advice myself. So think practically:
If you become a patient while taking care of a patient, who
will be the caregiver?

IN THE FALL of 1978, Margie noticed a large flat mass in
her right breast. It was not the pea or the egg she had been
hoping never to find, and because her breasts were large and
fibrous she assumed this was just a routine scare, a benign
boo. She briefly considered seeing our friend Dave Kinne—by
now chief of Memorial's breast service—but she was put off
by his reputation as an aggressive surgeon. She was afraid,
she said, that Dave would "just whip it right off." She had no
time for that now; I was in my first year of chemo, she was
trying to finish her novel, and both kids were in elementary
school.

She might have done nothing then if her mother wasn't
visiting when Margie discovered the mass. Margie showed it
to her. Ruby, who typically dismissed anything that wasn't
bleeding from an artery, looked serious and rolled her eyes.
That scared Margie enough to mention it to Tom Reynolds
during one of our pre-chemo kaffeeklatsches. He ordered her
to check it out. She made an appointment at the Strang Clinic
in downtown Manhattan.

In 1978, Strang was ahead of its time in head-to-toe cancer screening. Most people then didn't mention cancer, much
less take themselves in (as they did their cars) for periodic in-
spections. Furthermore, many doctors discouraged their patients from going to Strang. In that patronizingly learned way

that doctors of my generation dispensed medical journal statistics as well as medical convention hearsay, they spun the Clinic's specialization and technical focus into a negative question: Why would you want to be examined by doctors who don't know you as a human being and won't be involved in your care?

There was validity to that argument only if you were lucky enough to be in the care of a doctor who not only knew you as a human being but also had the expertise and machinery to check you out thoroughly.

The day Margie took her tests was that chemo Friday that the eager young radiologist thought he spotted a suspicious mass on my chest X-ray. By the time the doctors returned laughing about my "artifact," her own concerns had been shunted aside by my panic.

The following week, in a snowstorm, we went back to Strang for the results of her tests. A doctor she didn't much like said the mass was benign. Naturally, we were delighted. It may even have been true, right up until the spring of 1981, when Margie's local New Jersey gynecologist said the mass now felt different to her palpation and should be biopsied. In a chilling replay of my own first cancer, the gynecologist sent us to a local cancer surgeon, who made an appointment to operate in a local hospital.

Not that there is ever a good time for cancer, but tumors have a way of popping up when you are just too busy for them. Surprising how you find the time. Margie and I were both deep into new books, and although it was a risky financial stretch we had decided to buy land in the country and to build an addition to our split-level suburban house. My cancer had taught us—or we used it as an excuse—not to defer life-affirming gestures. Tomorrow is not promised.

My cancer had also taught us not to stick with local doctors. Dave Kinne was out of town, but my old friend Mark referred us to a courtly Fifth Avenue doctor, a lanky Yankee who sent Margie to the top mammogram expert in the city and then called her the next day to come in with me to review the results. He would not discuss them over the phone.

We would have been petrified by that meeting if Margie hadn't had a date to appear on Howard Cosell's radio show, "Speaking of Everything," to talk about her novel, which was just coming out in a paperback edition. Howard was an old friend, but Margie was not an experienced talk-show guest and we spent more time preparing for the meeting with Cosell than worrying about the meeting with the doctor, a blessing. Cosell was a wonderful interviewer, and the show went so well that we sailed into the doctor's office on a high that lasted until he told us that the mammogram was "suspicious," and that he was fairly sure the mass was malignant. Because of the large size of the lump, more than two centimeters, he advised a one-step procedure, a "wide excisional" biopsy that, if the tumor was indeed malignant, would continue on into a "modified radical," in which the breast and the lymph nodes under the arm would be removed.

As he explained in a reassuring baritone, this was fairly standard. The traditional Halsted radical mastectomy, developed in the 1890s at Johns Hopkins, in which the muscles of the breast and chest wall were removed, was now considered unnecessarily disfiguring—it didn't prolong life. And the lumpectomy-cum-radiation technique was still controversial.

Through it all, I took notes, tiny scribbles on a tiny pad, which I have still. On one sheet, above the doctor's name and address, is "Ridgewood Kitchens" and a telephone number. Below his name were the names of doctors at Mount Sinai and Memorial and "Cabinet Creations." Everyday life goes on. Even while we were shopping for doctors, we were shopping for our new kitchen.

My notes, I can tell, were purely functional. I had not yet begun the ostentatious notetaking on large pads that I later hoped would not only intimidate the medical-industrial complex but also keep my own motor running. I was fighting the creeping numbness, the natural inclination of my mind and body to shut down. Taking notes kept me in the game, although it didn't prevent a stony cold flower from growing and opening its heavy petals in my stomach. But taking notes has always helped me control panic, and taking notes shows doctors that you are paying attention, that their time is not wasted in explanation. The prime reason for taking notes, however, is simply to have an accurate record of what was said during what is so often a tense and hurried meeting. You will want to think about what was said, you will want to discuss it with others, perhaps including other doctors. You will be hearing words you don't understand, that you may want to look up later in a medical dictionary, and you will be hearing phrases about your heart valve or connective tissues or retina or spine that will need eventual explanation. Those notes will be the foundation on which you will build your own understanding of what is happening, the basis on which your decisions about your life, or the life of the person you are caring for, will be made. Some people even tape-record medical conversations, which is better.

Margie and I knew enough by then to know that we didn't have to make a decision on the spot. In the course of discussing options, Dave Kinne's name came up. The doctor graciously suggested we wait a day or so until Dave returned from vacation.

While we were more knowledgeable than we had been before August 1978—we did not necessarily think the word cancer was a death sentence—breast cancer scared us. It was more serious than testicular, a sneakier disease the doctors knew less about and for which they had less effective chemo.

Margie sobbed as we drove home from the doctor. She was somehow convinced she would die in six months or a year, and that she wouldn't see the kids grow up. Sam was almost thirteen then. Susannah was ten.

We told them right away, over a cold comfort dinner of delicatessen sandwiches and ice cream. Sam took it stoically. He was ready to pull her out of soft chairs as he had pulled me. Susannah's face twisted and turned red. She ran upstairs to cry. But she soon came back down, and we all talked some more and laughed and made plans. In retrospect, I think we did the right thing by telling them as much as we knew then; at that age they would have sensed that something was wrong, and their fantasies would have made it worse. And we let them be part of the solution, thinking of ways they could help out around the house, small ways for starters, which wouldn't disrupt their lives. Kids are practical survivors when given the chance. I remember a friend who described his upcoming open-heart surgery to his children, even going so far as to take off his shirt and sketch in charcoal the surgeon's incisions on his chest. The kids nodded seriously, then flipped a coin to see who would get to take Dad, after he came home from the hospital, to school for show and tell.

The night we told the kids about Margie's tumor was also the deadline to make a final decision about the windows in the proposed new bedroom, which would be built atop the new kitchen. Our original blueprints had small windows, to cut down on heating and air-conditioning costs. We had been swept along by the worthy ecological concerns of the man who drew the plans. But the architect who came to certify them took one look at the shimmering reservoir adjoining our property and began sketching in floor-to-ceiling picture windows. Didn't we want to wake up to that stunning water view? Suddenly, we did. Choosing the big windows was another life-affirming decision that we made at the borders of Malady. I am certainly not suggesting a bank-busting spree to counter every unwelcome diagnosis, but the lesson of those water-view windows—which gave us enormous pleasure for years—was one I wish I could be surer I would always follow. The phrase "Don't defer joy" probably sums up that lesson best.

Dave Kinne, steady and brisk, came back from vacation and began laying out the options in a reassuring monotone. It came down to lumpectomy versus mastectomy. We talked to other doctors, but we were eventually guided by his judgment that "You might do as well but you will never do better than a mastectomy." This was no time to take risks.

The operation went well. The pathologists found no cancer in the twenty-six nodes that Dave took out. Margie was quickly alert. We were both surprised that the operation wasn't so awful. The flip side of all the talk of mutilation and diminishment was the realization that the operation was mostly outside the body. It was an amputation, not an exploration of internal organs. And while Dave's aggressive reputation was justified, it was matched by his artistic skill. His scar is still one of the best in the business.

Naturally gregarious Margie began chatting up women on her floor. She never had the ballteam I did, but she didn't need it. Women are better than men at sharing information and feelings, and by then Memorial had groups in place for emotional counseling and physical rehab.

Margie found it helpful to be among people with the same disease, even if some were dying. Margie was no hospital rookie, although she had never been seriously ill; she had had three cesarean sections in a little more than four years, and knew something about recovering from surgery. The first C-section had been an emergency. The obstetrician discovered that our baby's umbilical cord was wound around her neck. She would be strangled during a normal delivery. Despite the operation, the baby died. It was terrible for both of us to be on the maternity floor while Margie recovered. We would walk corridors among cooing parents and grandparents and try to avoid looking at the bassinets of newborn babies. It was easy to understand why a woman might steal one.

The colleague's wife who had seemingly appeared to me in a pot haze in 1978 had been having her first baby at the same time in 1966 that we lost ours. When she found out that Margie was getting Jello and she wasn't, she threw a fit, raged through the halls screaming at nurses and invoking her connections. Eventually, she found out about the C-section and the baby's death, and was briefly contrite. Personalities are intensified under stressful circumstances, and being in a hospital rates high on the stress counter. Experienced patients cut slack for one another, and expect it themselves. Calm, firm, humane nurses seem to be the key to keeping the emotional heat down. Sedation helps, too.

It's too bad they can't also sedate visitors.

One immediately useful point I had learned from my own first trip to Malady was the importance of being something of a tour guide for the patient. I was particularly conscientious about keeping our own medical chart for Margie and riding herd on the day-trippers. I certainly took that role more seriously during her battle with cancer in 1981 than during the three C-sections, two of which turned out to be joyous celebrations. I might have been a bit too officious after Margie's mastectomy; nowadays I'd try to be more master of ceremonies and less security chief. But as much as family members and friends need to be reassured, the patient is the priority. And the patient's world is the reality.

The nurses and residents whom Margie liked were not necessarily my picks, and vice versa. We went back and forth about which of them was sexist, insecure, arrogant, patronizing, plain stupid. Ultimately, I learned to keep what I thought to myself, and certainly never, ever, express it to a person in white. This is an important rule in-country. If I thought the doctor or nurse was plain stupid, it would then become my job to gather more opinions or to discreetly check the labels on medicines and the clamps on IV drips. If I thought

Margie's room was dirty, I'd clean it up. Big deal. Save the noise for crises.

Roommates were like classmates or bunkmates or teammates, not for me to judge unless one screamed all night or had visitors who line-danced around the beds, in which case it would be my job to ask the nurses to intervene.

Margie was in Memorial for ten days, which would be rare now. There was some problem with wound drainage, but the length of time really had to do with unmanaged care. No one who was in charge seemed to be trying to contain costs, which was good for us. By the time Margie came home, she was strong and ready to resume ordinary life. These days, people have to try to complete their recoveries at home, with mixed results. If all goes well medically and there are attentive, low-key caregivers, home is probably a safer and less stressful environment for recovery. But complications can create a disruptive shuttle back and forth from home to hospital, and being tossed back into a demanding home while still weak may delay a recovery, even make it impossible. If there's a choice between home and hospital care, the best decision may not be a medical one but a kind of psycho-social-ecological one, preferably made by the patient and the primary caregiver, perhaps with the help of the wise nurse–clinician types who seem to be appearing at the more progressive hospitals.

WE KEPT LOOKING at kitchen sinks and cabinets while we shopped for the next medical procedure, which eventually came down to chemo or no chemo. Kinne, like Whitmore, was ahead of his time in advising "adjuvant" chemo as a mop-up after surgery even though there was no discernible spread. He was no macho cutter crowing, "I got it all, now go home and forget about it." Kinne said he was beginning to "lose" otherwise "clean" women and it bothered him; this was a man who had moved from heroic early transplant surgery to breast cancer because he wanted to watch patients grow old.

The cancer, according to my notes from Dave and from the oncologist, Thomas Hakes, was lobular, which meant it had arisen in the milk-producing glands of the breast, rather than the ducts. Margie's estrogen receptors were positive, which was good; statistically that meant less of a chance of recurrence. The tumor was three centimeters in circumference, fairly large, which was not good; statistically that meant more of a chance of recurrence. There had been cancerous spots elsewhere in the right breast, and while there was no node involvement, no obvious spread beyond the breast, that didn't mean cells hadn't been "shed" into the blood and lymphatic system. Of course, the immune system might kill them off before they grew strong and multiplied. We were told there was a 25 percent chance of recurrence, which chemo might reduce to 5 percent. There was also a lobular carcinoma in situ in the left breast, a precancerous condition that would not be treated now but could become an invasive cancer later. There were a lot of question marks in my notes.

Given the choice later, Margie would have had the chemo and a total mastectomy on the left side too. She remembered a nurse saying, "If it was me, I'd do it all."

At the time, however, we felt enough on the edge just going for the chemo, which was not routine then for women with no involved nodes. We talked to doctors at other hospitals (one oncologist was quickly deleted from our list when she labeled "Awful!" a floor of only breast cancer patients). But it was my experience, which had made Margie "braver" about cancer, that tipped the scales toward chemo. Our judgment was skewed by the success of chemo in treating my cancer. Chemotherapeutic drugs, discovered accidentally during studies of the World War I killer mustard gas, have fulfilled their early hype in only a few cancers, but one of the most dramatic successes was testicular.

Margie had six months of chemo, weekly doses of fluorouracil (better known as 5-FU), methotrexate, and vincristine, which was stopped because it caused tingling in her hands. We drove into the city from suburban New Jersey once a week for six months, a more pleasant commute than mine. Until the end, when there was some fatigue and stomach upset, she tolerated the chemicals well. She also had Leukeran, nine months of tamoxifen by mouth, and prednisone to "build me up and make me crazy," which it did.

Tom Reynolds called the protocol "covering the waterfront." With his usual bluntness, he added, "Chemo may not affect your survivability by one day, but it will keep you symptom-free until the cancer comes back in a whoooosh— and takes you pretty quickly."

BECOMING "The Cancer Couple" at a time when cancer was coming out of the closet should have led us into some active role, organizing groups, at least writing about it. How many married suburban couples with young children had experience as both patients and caregivers? To this day I'm not sure why we didn't use this experience to help others and make money for ourselves. We talked about it, but never got serious. Were we afraid of becoming too identified with the disease? Were we too dedicated to our own projects? Or was something else at work?

We were offered a sort of modern mom-and-pop ethics/ manners column by the *Washington Post Sunday Magazine*. It was enormously attractive to me; the money was good and the columns might lead to a book. I was very disappointed when I came back from Washington with the offer and Margie turned it down. She argued that because I now had a regular job at CBS, much of the research, the drudge work, would fall to her. This was true. I implied—maybe she inferred—that it was time for her to bring in some money. A rare squabble began. I backed off. This was a touchy area that we had never resolved in almost twenty years. I still resented her quitting the *Times* while we were living together but before we were married. She quit while I was away on Army reserve duty, so there was no chance for discussion. She said that the job, staff editor in the women's section, was going nowhere, and that she didn't think she could handle such a demanding job and our relationship at the same time. Not only did we lose her salary, but also her independence. I felt trapped, especially when she had to stop paying rent on her old apartment.

It was not something I thought about much after we got married in 1966. And once the kids came, it was history. But by the early eighties, I thought it was history worth studying, especially in the climate of the women's movement, which Margie had embraced. There were plenty of other early-middle-aged couples trying to reconcile a fifties' mindset with the opportunities and demands of so-called liberation. They would be the core audience for our *Post* column. Editor Ben Bradlee had been easy to convince, especially since my friend Jay Lovinger, the magazine's editor, had dreamed up the column. But I couldn't convince Margie.

Sometimes I wonder if the seed of our marriage's breakup was planted before we ever got married, when she quit. And I wonder what would have happened if we had done the column together and become closer through the effort and its possible success. Television was already pulling us apart. I was traveling often as a correspondent for "Sunday Morning with Charles Kuralt." Margie had little interest in TV, and some contempt for it. She was working on her next novel. So we never got to explore all that history, certainly not as it pertained to us.

When we met at the *Times* in 1963, our mindset assumed that my work and ambitions would take precedence over hers. Some of it was conditioning and some of it was practical. Although I was six years younger, I was far more advanced in my career than she was in hers, and as a young man, all else being equal, I could make far more money than a young woman could.

After Margie quit work in 1964, two years before we married, I became our total support. Despite my resentment at not being consulted, I was proud that I could carry the financial load alone. The messages I sent out were mixed, confusing to both of us. Part of me wanted a nonworking woman at home. My mother was a teacher and she worked until I was seven, when my sister was born. I remembered being taken care of by bored young women who gossiped in the park with other babysitters. The mid-sixties were already toward the end of the postwar, middle-class, split-level nuclear family togetherness cycle. Within ten years, women were expected to get out and hunt too, and men were chided if they weren't willing to tend the home fires.

The so-called "liberated man" was supposed to not only share in household and childrearing duties so the new woman could express herself professionally, but also get in touch with his feminine side, the nurturing, caring, intuitive parts of his psyche, so he could do just as good a job around the home as the woman, and do it as a full self-starting partner rather than a grudging helper.

Yet if he did—and very few of us really did—the woman might tend to feel displaced. After all, it was unlikely she was making as much money as he was, or getting the same kind of on-the-job reinforcement and satisfaction.

If this seems complicated—it reads complicated to me as I write it now—you can imagine the adjustment, the constant tacking and trimming, that living it demanded. Margie and I had an enormous advantage over many other couples at first; I was working primarily at home in those years, and she not only understood my work, but also was supportive of it and editorially helpful. And I was enthusiastic about feminism, not so much as a redress for old grievances but as a possible liberation for men—if women could choose to work and receive equivalent pay, there would be more options for men like me who might want to step out of the race to take a flyer on a project, like a book or a movie. Margie was very active in *New Directions for Women*, a now-defunct national feminist newspaper, as well as the National Organization for Women and a local women's group called Northern Valley Women for Today (NOVA).

Margie and I had worked out a schedule of sorts; we alternated years in which one or the other was the parent-in-charge, getting up at night to answer a child's cry and taking the kids to and from school, the doctor, Brownies, soccer, Little League. It was never hard-and-fast, or truly equal. I'd get an out-of-town assignment or need to make a meeting. Margie filled in for me far more often than I did for her, but the schedule gave her more time to write and attend feminist meetings and it enriched my life. I loved being around Sam and Susannah. The years after I was sick might have had an added poignancy or urgency for me—I'm simply not sure—but just watching kids grow and having a potter's hand in shaping that growth is as thrilling and creative (and, yes, sometimes as frustrating and boring) as anything else I could do. Those years were also critical to my relationship with the kids later, when life got even more complicated. We had logged *quantitative* time, we had shared memories, we could speak openly. Not that everything went smoothly, but there was, I think, a basic sense we all had that we could quarrel and still come together again.

The most profound thing I learned from those years was this: Whoever is responsible is the mom. When it was my year to get up, I would hear Sam or Susannah call out in the middle of the night, and Margie wouldn't; also vice versa. So much for biological imperatives.

If you think such earned wisdom makes life simpler, you weren't around in the seventies and eighties trying to grow out of a fifties sensibility. But it did make caregiving easier and more natural. I had chauffeured, cooked meals, made beds, run errands when nobody was sick. Doing it while Margie recovered didn't seem overwhelming. I was still primarily working at home, pretty much in charge of my own schedule. And it wasn't some big gender issue. We had practiced for this. Again, it was not quite equal; I had much less to do for her journey than she did for mine.

Margie was a good patient, spirited, positive, intent on getting back to everyday life quickly, so my insights into caregiving then were somewhat abstract. I wasn't facing the endless grind of a long-term chronic disease or the hopelessness of a terminal journey. Money was not an issue at the time, since insurance covered most everything. Margie was not working and I was able to keep writing, but I could see how an illness could suck savings, energy, possibility, life itself into a black hole. I could imagine an exhausted, overwrought caregiver praying for relief. Would he become so desperate he would withhold a lifesaving procedure or actually press a pillow to a patient's face until breathing stopped? Or do it psychologically, administering a guilt-drip until the patient found a way to kill himself?

It was some years later that I got a greater insight into heavy-duty caregiving through my friends Seth and Orren Gelblum. Their second daughter, Morgan, was born with

Canavan's disease, a rare, fatal, neurological degeneration that mostly strikes children of Eastern European Jewish ancestry. She seemed healthy at birth, but by four months she appeared to be developing slowly. At eight months, she seemed to have stopped. Because of the obscurity of the disease, she was not diagnosed until she was fifteen months old.

At seven, when she was a smiling, beatific presence at a dinner party I attended, she had the neurological capacity of an infant; she never even crawled. She had teeth but couldn't chew food. Because she had difficulty swallowing, she was fed baby food. Her sight was fading. Her prognosis was openly discussed in the noisy living room.

"I know she is going to die," said Seth that night, rolling Morgan around his football lineman's shoulders, "and I've learned that you can hold two contradictory emotions, sadness and relief. At the moment though, when I think about it, and I do every day, it's just sadness. Orren doesn't think about it. I don't think she has the time."

Despite Medicaid-funded home care, Morgan's daily life—the preparation for school (she was bussed to special-education classes in Manhattan), the frequent doctors' appointments, the occasional hospital stays after seizures, the daily medications, the changing and feeding—was an awesome grind.

"But there's an upside, too," said Orren. "Morgan brings great joy, she is a happy, responsive spirit and she is not emotionally demanding. She doesn't mind if Madeleine or Aidan sits on my lap. I think the grandparents took it even harder, they only saw the downside. My mother thought it was a crime that people had to go through this."

Orren's mother, Eileen Alperstein, now deceased, was a board member of Planned Parenthood and one of the early engines of the Canavan Foundation. The family found other parents and grandparents with Canavan kids and formed an association that raised money not only for research but to develop a simple blood-test that would identify carriers of the disease. In this case, the caregivers may actually have a hand in lowering the disease's incidence, if not eventually eradicating it.

Morgan died at seven, and there was relief and sadness. The Gelblums had made her part of the family. Three-year-old Aidan somehow included her in his living-room football games, if only by making her wheelchair a goalpost, and eleven-year-old Madeleine discussed her homework with Morgan, even if she could only smile. But there was reality, too.

"Would we have aborted her if we had known?" Orren paused, not so much for thought but out of respect for the question. "Yes."

TWO WEEKS AFTER the operation, Margie was swimming again. Amazing. She was also parading. Never overly modest in the locker room, Margie was now marching with a towel casually thrown over a shoulder or wrapped around her waist, her one-breasted chest bared. I listened to her triumphant reports of women shocked or liberated or indignant at her defiant demonstrations.

There were women who ducked and cowered in the locker room when they saw her coming, women upset that young girls were exposed to this exposure. Margie had an answer.

"It's part of being a feminist," she would say. "What's the crime? Let people see it. This was kept from us; let's know it happens, that it's not so awful, that you can live a full life, play golf, make love, swim in the pool, work out. Let's demystify breast cancer."

Such sentiments were cropping up in feminist journals of the time, along with arty photographs of women who had

had breasts removed. Some had flowers tattooed on their chests, the petals growing out of the scar/stems. It seemed bold and whimsical to us at the time, a positive gesture.

But some people were deeply offended, including a supposedly progressive, nature-loving network television executive producer whose wife had just had a mastectomy. He scowled at the poster of an attractive, naked, middle-aged, one-breasted woman I gave him. He would never show his wife such pornography, he said. I thought he was going to tear up the poster. When I told Margie, she shrugged; he was part of the problem. I began to regard him differently after that. Was he withholding information just from his wife to keep her in check, or was this the true prism through which he decided which stories—including my stories!—got on the air?

Margie's inspiration was a tall, broad-shouldered young woman, perhaps nineteen or twenty, who also swam in her pool. One leg had been amputated above the knee. She had dropped out of an Ivy League college to battle sarcoma. She would swing into the pool area on crutches, drop them, and hop the rest of the way to the diving platform. She had a great stroke; she was an athlete if not a competitive swimmer. When she disappeared, we hoped her rehab was over and that she had gone back to school. We didn't want to consider the alternative.

But people were put off by that young woman's presence. Children shouldn't have to see this, they said. It was too scary, too real. People who weren't perfect should be hidden.

That's what Margie was protesting in the locker room, that small-minded attitude that can make the trip back home from Malady even more difficult for people who have been visibly changed. We often return from Malady with big scars, missing parts, in wheelchairs, speaking haltingly. Strokes, osteoporosis, multiple sclerosis, lupus, heart disease—the list goes on and on—leave their marks. In the summer of 1993, a topless photograph of the artist Matuschka, whom Margie knew, appeared on the cover of the *New York Times Magazine*. There was a mastectomy scar where her right breast had been. Many people wrote to the *Times* complaining that the picture was distasteful. But many, many more (Susannah briefly worked for Matuschka during this period and saw the mail) wrote and called to say "Thank you."

One of the most inspiring of Malady travelers has been Muhammad Ali, whose life with Parkinson's disease has been as public as was his life as a boxer, entertainer, and political and religious speaker. Trembling yet unself-conscious, he lit the Olympic flame in Atlanta in 1996, demonstrating that the only shame in disability is the shame of those who would hide it or discriminate against it.

The year before, during an interview with George Foreman, I asked the former boxing champion how he felt about Ali's diminished condition. His answer took my breath away.

"When you look at Muhammad Ali," said Foreman, smiling, "you think about veterans of World War II, the big war. It was really a great war, fought for something special. And when you're sitting in an office with them and they happen to take off a leg and say, 'Look what happened to me,' or take out an eye, 'Look what happened to me in that war,' it's a thing of pride. Muhammad felt like he did something more than box. He made a lot of people feel good about themselves."

Ali's most important lasting contribution, far beyond boxing, even beyond his political stands, may be how he made a lot of people feel good about themselves after a hard, even disfiguring, journey through Malady.

IN 1983, Margie wrote the following for *New Directions for Women:*

The day two and a half years ago when it seemed certain the lump in my breast was cancerous I had lunch with a trim, smartly dressed woman in her mid-60s who in the preceding eight years had a breast removed, seen her husband die of cancer, had her other breast removed and remarried. "Remember," she said in an effort to cheer me up, "it's on the outside. The surgery is on the outside."

Outside, inside, this woman is mad, I thought. Losing a breast is the worst thing that can happen to a woman. I'd been conditioned to believe that since I was a girl. Losing a breast disfigures a woman, desexes a woman. A woman without a breast is like a bicycle without a wheel. Of all the horrors that cancer invokes, losing a breast seemed especially horrible. Even this woman, I knew, had been upset immediately after her mastectomies. How could she be so chipper now? She must be truly mad.

But I soon learned that she wasn't mad at all. It was the cancer that was important, not the breast or lack of it. After the early pain of surgery and the strain of physical exercise there was a period when I had to get used to my different body, my "changed landscape," as Audre Lorde calls it. Though the surgery wasn't all on the outside—I had nodes removed—I quickly saw that my main concerns were how best to deal with the cancer, what course of treatment to pursue, what kind of prosthesis, if any, to buy, which was the most comfortable position for sleep, where to have pockets sewn in my bathing suit.

It's true I missed the erotic pleasure from the absent breast and my arm was weaker and vulnerable to lymphedema, a painful and ugly swelling, but my life was not appreciably different. My prognosis is good, I have other erotic areas, and sooner than I would have ever dreamed I was going full tilt. I still wondered why so much that had been written about breast cancer seemed to sidestep meaningful discussion of the disease itself and concentrated instead on the presumed psychological trauma special to having a breast removed. What was all the noise about, I wondered, confident that it was all in the past, that in the '80s it would no longer be automatically assumed that living without a breast or two was the worst that could happen to a woman.

And for awhile it seemed true. There seemed to be fewer articles about the marvels of prosthesis with "real looking" nipples and the clever nighties and sleeping bras we can wear. There was more about the latest drug and hormone treatments and the relationship of the diet to cancer.

Then reconstructive surgery became the rage. Advances in the technique, coverage by hospital insurance, and a barrage of books and articles contributed to the excitement. Women who didn't feel like women after mastectomies could feel whole again, and women who were afraid to have their breasts examined could now seek medical attention because they knew they could have the prosthesis under their skin.

The first thing a doctor told a young friend after she learned she had breast cancer was that she was a perfect candidate for reconstructive surgery. "I wanted to talk about my chances," she told me, still indignant, "and they thought all I wanted to hear was that I could get some silicone put inside me."

Still the emphasis on the breast and not the disease. I thought about the women I know who had mastectomies and the only common denominator I found among them—whether they opted for reconstructive surgery or not—is their concern about their life, their health, their survival rate. They worry more about their nodes than their nipples. The same concerns that any rational person with a serious cancer would have. Why then, I wondered, are we still being trivialized in public print and private medical offices? Why do editors and doctors alike think the first thing we want to hear is we can have silicone inside our skin to simulate a breast? Or that the trend away from mastectomies toward lumpectomies is the good news we've all been waiting for?

Lumpectomy patients rated their husbands' sexual behavior as enhanced after surgery, compared to mastectomy patients, who felt that their husbands' sexual behavior showed a decline, according to a recent book. The author shouts the good news—no more mastectomies. To me, the good news would be no more breast cancer or better survival rates.

When procedures like lumpectomy plus radiation and/or chemotherapy become the norm in treating most breast cancers, we can all cheer. And from the data accumulating from current large-scale studies, it looks like that day is getting closer. But before we go overboard, let's remember we're talking about cancer and not a facelift.

While I tended to agree politically with Margie, our personal approaches to our diseases were different. My healing process was about rushing through recovery to get back to ordinary life, or as close to what had come before as was possible. Let's get on with it. She worked her way back slowly, through a grieving process. I thought she left no thought or emotion unturned or unexpressed, that she sometimes wallowed self-indulgently. She felt I sometimes refused to face issues and left them unresolved. We had different emotional styles and we probably should have worked harder at accommodating the differences. We were better during crises at giving each other slack than during everyday life. While I've come to believe that whatever works for someone is right, I also think that I might have done better as patient and person by slowing down that rush back to business as usual and trying to more fully understand what I was going through while I was going through it.

SEVEN YEARS after he pulled me out of soft chairs, Sam wrote a one-act play set in a generic hospital chemo waiting room. He was a counselor at summer camp between his junior and senior years in high school, and he wrote the play in one night. I don't know how he managed to capture the chaotic edginess of patients and caregivers or to find as good a metaphor for cancer and its treatment as I have ever read.

In the play, a kid with cancer waiting for his chemo warns about a time "when you don't give a shit anymore . . . when you realize the poison they're shooting into your body might be worse than anything that could grow inside you . . . when you start to feel like everybody's throwing all kinds of shit at you, maybe not even to help you."

Another teenage patient says it reminds him of a vicious schoolyard game called "Bombardment."

The two boys reminisce about the game. Kids peg big red rubber balls at one another. They leap and twist and dodge to avoid the whizzing balls. If you're hit, you're out of the game. The winner is the last one standing.

I was proud of Sam's talent and glad someone in the family had gotten something literary out of the experience. But as cancer came out of the closet in the eighties, I slipped out of the room. I just wanted to get past it, come home from Malady and never go there again.

PART TWO

Sophisticated Travelers

6

I WAS OFFICIALLY declared cured in 1990 by the ultimate authority: a life insurance company. I was worth betting on again. After twelve years of being turned down for coverage (and, although I didn't find out for years, a TV staff position) because of my cancer history, I got a $200,000 policy.

The insurance company didn't even seem all that interested in my cancer history (although I needed to get a doctor to send a No Evidence of Disease letter). Once I passed my blood test, the company was happy to take my money and I was happy to believe their prognosis.

Cured!

Of course, that's a word I never use, and don't really believe in. "The cancer is in remission" sounds okay, although NED is good enough for me. Maybe I'm being superstitious and maybe I'm being scientific. Some people think there are always sneaky little assassin cells lurking in your body that are picked off by the snipers of the immune system until one day the defenses are down and a rogue cell slips in to start a new Murder Inc. franchise. I didn't visualize this scenario every single day, but it did recur from time to time. It was part of The Dread, which no serious visitor to Malady ever escapes.

In my case, the symptoms of The Dread were dry mouth, loose bowels, a toothache in my gut, worst of all a numbness, a physical and psychic paralysis that could strap me to a chair for hours, thoughtless, staring, Greg-like, every time I felt a strange pain, sweated in the night, was faced with an unexplained marker in a blood test or a shadow in an X-ray. Or thought a doctor or technician had glanced at me with narrowed eyes. Friends of mine who have had heart attacks get symptoms of The Dread from muscle aches in the chest, friends with Crohn's disease get them from an abdominal cramp.

Sometimes The Dread would just come and I wouldn't even know why. It would arrive with its own flashbacks: The swashbuckling surgeon pokes my tumor and chuckles to his apprentice, "Looks suspicious to me, let's go in there"; a nurse merrily shouts "Sharp stick!" as she injects me, and nausea scratches my throat as I recall the chilly prickle when a chemo bubble slides out of a silver needle to go rafting in my veins.

Once contracted, The Dread may be incurable, which doesn't mean it can't vanish for so long that you think you are free of it. But be aware that it does come back, and that it merely means you're scared again—it doesn't mean you are sick again. Not to compare myself to others who have suffered far, far more, but I do suspect that The Dread is similar to what Holocaust survivors, combat veterans, rape victims feel. The Dread is not cloudy and impressionistic like a fear of the unknown; it is intense and precise because you have felt the shape of what scares you.

When I could physically force myself up and moving, I could chase The Dread, which was most overpowering and frequent during those first few years after the initial diagnosis, when recurrence was most likely and when every lump in the night seemed to threaten cancer again. It came more often in the morning than the night, and pinned me to the bed. But getting out of bed, which sometimes felt like breaking out of a cage, was always a great first step to overcoming The

Dread. Movement was the key—out of bed, into the shower, out of the house, a brisk walk around the block, and it was gone. After I got my $200,000 death policy, I thought it was gone forever.

BY 1990, MY LIFE was entirely different. The policy was part of the divorce settlement. Marriages often break up from the stresses of illness, but I think that fighting the diseases together, as well as raising the children together, bound us longer. I sometimes wonder if the "empowerment" that Margie felt from taking charge while I was down contributed to changes in our relationship that eventually pulled us apart. We talked about it later, but never got very far. We also wondered about the sense of vulnerability I felt, the sense of mortality. Cancer was not the only factor in the breakup, but I'm sure it played a role. My lack of introspection and refusal to talk things through is a reason we will never be sure just how much it meant. I'm still not comfortable talking about the divorce.

In 1982, a year after Margie's cancer, I was offered a job as sports essayist for the best program on television, CBS's "Sunday Morning with Charles Kuralt." I had never thought of myself as a TV correspondent—too chubby, non-network hair, a New York accent—but they caught me between books with a nice enough offer. The people were congenial. After eleven years working mostly at home, an experience intensified by being a patient and a caregiver, getting out in the world seemed very attractive. The kids were now fourteen and eleven, a lot less interested in hanging out with me, so playmates were harder to find. And because I did not then feel emotionally invested in television, I thought I couldn't fail. I didn't mind doing sports again, since the "Sunday Morning" take on sports was anything but hard-core. I figured I would stay for the summer and get inside material and local color for another book. Maybe I would rewrite that thriller in the bottom drawer, with a television background.

I stayed at CBS for four happy, busy years, until I began to feel underpaid for such a TV star, jowls and all. My salary was doubled at NBC, where I appeared on nightly news shows and was busy and unhappy for two years. Then the wheel of fortune stopped on my number; a new nightly public affairs show on the local PBS station, WNET-13, was looking for a host with a New York sensibility and accent, jowls and non-network hair please apply. It was called "The Eleventh Hour," and it plunged me into a world of pols, celebs, cops, grassroots organizers, artists. It was intense and thrilling. One night Bishop Tutu, the next night Donald Trump, then a crack dealer, the mayor, an historian, the jazz musician Max Roach, Susan Sarandon ("Pronounced like 'abandon,' " she whispered). We won a lot of Emmys and were canceled after two seasons. Television.

IN EARLY 1991, The Dread recurred in a whooosh. I felt a lump on the remaining testicle.

The first time, my entire right testicle had swelled because the tumor was inside the gland, which I later found out was the less typical symptom. This time, I felt a hard little pea on the outside of the testicle, a more classic tumor. But the pea seemed part of a tangle of tubes and strands, varicose veins, and seminal ducts that felt as though they were all coming out of my testicle, that old linguine effect. My scrotal sac felt like a small bag of cooked pasta. I was scared but not totally convinced this was déjà vu all over again. But I did arm myself with tumor humor. The notation for January 29 on my calendar was "Going Nuts?"

I called Memorial. As an alumnus, even though no one in the urology department knew me any more, I got an appointment for the following week. It was five days of The Dread, of numbness and flashbacks, of thinking about castration and the end of manhood.

I kept remembering a "Sunday Morning" producer, Bill Moran, who would say to me, whenever I stepped into the recording booth for a voiceover, "Hairy balls now, let's hear hairy Walter Cronkite balls." My voice was thin—it didn't punch through without effort—so we would pretend this super-manliness.

I remembered the all-pervasive metaphor: Admire the guy with big balls, brass balls; forget him, he's got no balls; it's balls-to-the-wall time; show some balls; we'll find out now who has balls. There were women with balls, which made them honorary men.

I thought of a fellow writer whose doctors told him that castration—a double orchiectomy—was the only way to halt the spread of his prostate cancer. He didn't want the operation, but somehow they did it anyway, and he died anyway, muttering, "They took my balls, they took my balls."

I thought of Hemingway's Jake Barnes, narrator of *The Sun Also Rises,* who had, according to the Italian colonel, "given more than your life." A college professor had said that Jake, like Huck Finn, represented the observer as outsider, Jake because he had lost his manhood, the preadolescent Huck because he hadn't gotten it yet.

In 1978 and again in 1981, when Margie was diagnosed, I had thought primarily about surviving cancer, not about loss of a body part. In fact, Margie and I had talked at great length about how the media's obsession with breasts had skewed the coverage of breast cancer, often concentrating on women's fears of sexual, cosmetic, and emotional impairment rather than on fears of death and on the need for more research. But this time around, knowing I could live with cancer, I wondered if I could live without testicles.

After the operations in 1978—the orchiectomy and the retroperitoneal node dissection—it was several months before I was sexually active again. Even more than the surgeries, it was the chemo that suppressed desire. It's very hard to feel sexy and nauseated at the same time. The bigger operation, the node dissection, had damaged or numbed some nerves and I was left with "retrograde" or dry ejaculations, in which the semen flowed backward into the bladder during orgasm and was discharged with urine. This caused infertility, but had no effect on sexual performance or sensation. For a while, I did think that my orgasm felt different, less powerful but longer-lasting. Once I got over being frightened by the change itself, I rather liked it, and eventually missed it when everything returned to normal.

But this was going to be different. I could not imagine a positive side. For five days in early 1991, dry-mouthed, loose-boweled, constantly having to push myself out of the numbness, I tried to psych myself for a rematch with The Beast (contra Sontag, to be sure, but thinking about it in those mythic terms was helpful then, gave me a spurt of hero juice). I told myself that I was older this time, which would make my medical recovery more difficult, but my kids were older, which would be emotionally easier. I was in a happy, sexually satisfying relationship, so there would be much to lose; yet there would still be a relaxed atmosphere in which to explore alternatives.

The night before I called Memorial for the appointment, I shook The Dread long enough to take Margie to her favorite opera, *The Magic Flute*. We were by then legally separated and had made the first steps toward re-establishing a friendship that wasn't based only on the kids or financial matters. After twenty-five years, there was plenty to talk about. I wanted to mention my testicle, but I didn't. Was I shy, was it more intimate than I wanted to be? I was living with someone else, someone I would soon marry. But Margie would have been helpful, smart about it.

It's too bad we didn't start talking cancer again, because she was going through the beginnings of her own rematch, although she didn't know it yet. Maybe if I had started that conversation, she would have told me about the pains in her back and maybe I would have urged her to get a bone scan then. She attributed those pains to being thrown off-balance by her heavy left breast. She talked to her internist at Memorial about having the breast removed, but the doctor, a woman, thought it was "too radical" and suggested reconstructive surgery. The left breast could be made smaller and a matching right breast created with silicone.

Should the doctor have ordered a bone scan right then? Would that have led to radiation and chemo that might have killed the multiplying rogue cells?

But we didn't talk cancer on the night of *The Magic Flute* and I went home to roam through thirty years of calendars, almost 11,000 days, each with its own square on which I'd noted weight, exercise, pages written, leaves raked, cars taken for maintenance, school plays attended, kids' sicknesses, friends, movies, plays seen. I searched for trends, curves, signals in my life leading up to the 1978 cancer that could be matched with parallel tracks leading up to an answer in 1991. Was there a code to be cracked?

Friends my age had started dying—the writer Pete Axthelm from years of drug and alcohol abuse, producer Lee Reichenthal after an unusually long battle with pancreatic cancer, and, most traumatically for me, my tennis partner, the economics professor Alfred Eichner, who had fallen dead after a racketball game. More than the others, Al's death at fifty had reminded me of my own intimations of mortality. It was his death in the winter of 1988 while I was covering the Calgary Olympics that convinced me to change my life, to move on, to leave Margie. I had just turned fifty.

I am a sucker for portents and symbols and omens. Why else in 1991 was I rereading, and relishing, Mary Renault's *The Persian Boy*, who was brutally castrated at eleven?

I was in the midst of writing *The Chemo Kid*.

I had just accepted an offer from Carey Winfrey to write a column for *American Health* magazine. Carey had offered me the assurance that at my age enough bad things would happen to fill one thousand words a month for years. We had both chuckled at that, Carey more heartily.

And I was in serious negotiations to return to the *Times* after twenty years, which had felt sometimes like liberation and sometimes like exile. My life was taking a major turn. It also seemed as though it was turning back. To cancer?

So I feverishly scoured the calendars that night looking for seven-year cycles, health-and-sickness cycles, good-year–bad-year cycles. Was there an event that had opened the immune gates to the barbarian cells starting that first cancer in 1978—the death of the baby in 1966, the failure of my Big Novel, *Liberty Two*, in 1972, the loss of my *New York Post* cityside column in 1977 because Rupert Murdoch didn't like the way I was writing about his favorite politicians? Margie and I, who together pooh-poohed such stress-point theories of cancer, liked to joke about suing Murdoch or the critic who had savaged *Hot Type* for cancer damages.

But now I wondered if a second cancer was growing in response to the breakup of my marriage, to the cancellation of my talk show.

I report this crazy thinking—and I do think it is crazy thinking—because it is common and understandable, an attempt to find a pattern in chaos, the medical equivalent of wanting to believe that an assassination was part of a conspiracy rather than an act of random violence.

I truly believe that most of our heart attacks, strokes, and cancers are natural acts of random violence. An immune system going mad is a personal tornado. Sure, we could make ourselves healthier through diet, exercise, and stress reduction (and a wiser choice of the genes we inherit), but when illness does strike, unless it is, say, cancer in a smoker's lung, it can rarely be precisely attributed to how one lived a life, much less such vague emotional states as optimism or sociability.

But that's just what I think and has nothing to do with how I *feel*. The Dread settled in like an island fog. I was going under the knife again. This time the stakes were higher.

My girlfriend—now wife—Kathy was out of town, in the critical stages of a TV shoot. I didn't want to dump it all out on her over the phone. What a guy. So I went down to St. Petersburg to dump it out in person. I was tense and whiny but it helped. Me.

THE WAITING ROOM on the urological floor at Memorial hadn't changed in thirteen years, still drab and crowded with men in their sixties and seventies with troublesome prostates and bladders, an occasional young man with his mother. A testicular? Should I talk to him, offer him encouragement? But I was no encouragement now, and my information was probably out of date.

It was indeed. The nurse who drew my blood had been at Memorial for eighteen years. I ran down the roster of my old doctors—all had retired or moved on. Treatments are "more humane now," she told me, shorter, more intense blasts of chemo under sedation in the hospital. She kept stabbing the big vein in the crook of my right arm, but nothing came out. It was still dead from chemo. I asked her what veins they would use this time—thigh, neck, between my toes?—but she pretended not to hear.

Later, after she struck blood in my hand and left, I wrote it all down on a small, unintimidating notepad. Good stuff for the book I hadn't written the first time.

The examining room was still small and chilly. There was blood in the toilet. I was naked. Through the dusty window I could see a sunny winter day and hear children yelling in a playground. Too obvious for the book. The TV movie? I gave myself a self-conscious chuckle. Love that 'tude, Bobby.

The Surgeon and his younger associate knocked before they entered. They were both brownish men, Indian and Cambodian, cheerful but reserved, brisk pros, no swash-bucklers. They poked and squeezed and seemed faintly disappointed. A mass all right, but they didn't think it was malignant. Could be epididymitis. Their expression conveyed vaguely that I had let them down. The blood still had to be analyzed for markers, and a sonogram might yet spot a whisper of disease. We would meet again in three weeks.

I tried to press them on the worst-case scenario. What would it mean, an empty sac? How would it affect my energy, my appearance, my general health? Would testosterone replacement help?

You're getting ahead of the story, they said.

Maybe so, I said, but we are talking about the metaphor for my manhood. In a country where sex is still considered the best way to sell beer, lose weight, and make friends, I told them, losing your erection is like losing your credit cards. Will I be losing my credit cards?

They chuckled patronizingly. Let's wait and see. Come back in three weeks. I didn't like the senior surgeon; he seemed sweet and vague, too wishy-washy. He never looked directly at me. Perhaps it was cultural. Perhaps he was impatient because I was wasting his time. There were people in that waiting room with . . . cancer.

The next three weeks slid by more easily than the previous five days. The Dread made its morning appearance, but most of the time I managed to tear off that blanket of depression just by jumping out of bed.

I wrote about The Dread for my first *American Health* column. See, said editor Carey, I was counting on bad things happening to good writers. The *Times* negotiations heated up. I did a number of interviews for a ten-hour documentary on Muhammad Ali, my *Times* touchstone. Everyday life rolled on.

The night before the sonogram, I called my friend Roger Sims, a former TV colleague, a smart, gentle man, but also a dude with 'tude shaped by being black and hardened in Vietnam.

"Waaaal, Bobby," he rumbled over the phone from a Seattle suburb, "let's make a deal. You give me one of your kidneys, I'll give you one of my balls."

Tumor humor. We riffed for a while on what it would be like for me with one of his testicles. He said he couldn't promise better sex, but I'd certainly have more appreciation for jazz. I might even remember how to fly an Air Force jet. I felt better.

A friend like Roger can make a big difference in a critical time, especially if your friend has been there and is willing to talk openly and—more important—allow you to talk openly. Too many conversations, even with close, loving people, require patients to pull their punches, downplay their fears. You need listeners who will let you laugh or cry. Cherish such friends. Often, they are not even your closest friends or relatives. Since he moved West, I see Roger only every few years, although we talk often on the phone.

Roger is my age, and has been a diabetic since his pancreas failed in 1971. He became insulin-dependent. He has dealt with impotence and a penile implant, gangrene, minor strokes, laser eye surgery to repair retinal damage, and, since his kidneys failed, thrice-weekly, six-hour sessions with a dialysis machine that often leave him exhausted. At the time I was worried about losing a second testicle, he was waiting for a kidney transplant.

When his kidney call finally came—at six on a Sunday morning—he'd been waiting more than two years. The transplant coordinator explained that they weren't yet absolutely sure Roger and the kidney were a match—they were waiting for the result of one more blood test—but if it was a go the organ would be transplanted that evening.

He packed in a few minutes, then took a few minutes more to figure out the correct number of socks to pull over the stump of his left leg. Most of the leg below the knee had been amputated less than five months earlier to halt a raging infection, and the swollen stump was still in the process of shrinking into the socket of the prosthesis. The thickness of the socks helps distribute the weight around the rim of the socket; it's important not to bear down directly on the tip of the stump, especially if you are 6 feet 6 inches tall and weigh 240 pounds, as does Roger. When the stump was at its thickest, right after the amputation, a one-ply sock was enough. Dressing for the hospital, Roger pulled on several socks, totaling six ply.

The drive to the Swedish Hospital Medical Center in Seattle took more than the usual twenty-five minutes because of a heavy fog and because Roger was still teaching his prosthesis to come up slowly on the clutch. But by 7:45 a.m. he was in his room, listening to his surgeon, Dr. William H. Marks, explain that unless the match was complete, there was a risk the "kidney would die, just turn black from the antibody."

"Black's okay with me," said Roger. Dr. Marks laughed and left.

Roger called me that afternoon. He would know in about three hours. "I'm not allowing myself to get excited," he said. But he must have been waving his arms because the alarm on the dialysis machine went off twice while we talked.

"If I don't call you back tonight," he said, "that means they're operating on me."

We didn't talk again until Monday midnight. He was still groggy, but he had a new kidney, from an adolescent in Alaska. It might take up to two weeks to be sure it would work, he said, but the five-hour operation had gone well and although the kidney hadn't kicked in yet, everyone was optimistic.

The optimism grew for the ten days he was in the hospital. The new kidney had been attached to his dead left kidney and it bulged out through his skin.

"Rub it, you two have to get to know each other," said Dr. Marks, and Roger did, while wondering how the youngster had died, why that youngster's family had donated the organ. There are an estimated 28,000 Americans waiting for a kidney, but despite the tragic abundance of potential donors—the otherwise healthy young victims of violent death—the supply of organs is far below the demand.

Roger went home after ten days. He wasn't prepared for the fatigue. He had hoped to keep up his walking regimen to further toughen and compress his stump, but even the 200 yards to the mailbox was a marathon. Stairs were a problem. Still, he had gotten the socks up to thirteen ply. "Stump used to look like a big fat salami," he said, "and now it's a worn-down eraser on a pencil."

He was taking fifteen different drugs every morning and seven different drugs every night, which added up to several dozen pills and a bill of $819 a month. Medicare would pay the bill for a year as part of his disability benefits.

Two weeks almost to the hour after he had heard a nurse shout, "It's a match, Roger, let's rumble!" he was sounding alternately thoughtful and angry, a healthy sign.

He was thoughtful about the little kidney pumping away. He felt "a little guilty" that he was alive and the adolescent from Alaska was not. While the transplant team would give him no further information about his donor, they promised to forward a letter to the family. But what should I say, Roger wondered, wouldn't I just be satisfying my own curiosity? How can I ever thank them enough? The sensitive side of Roger struggled with a letter to grieving parents. The tough side of Roger was angry at the politicians and media pundits debating health care on TV.

"I feel such rage at those inside-the-Beltway guys; they all have their insurance and they talk about health care as if it's some game. Their attitude seems to be, 'I'd like my side to win this game, but if we don't, well, okay, we're all men of good will here and the ship of state will sail on.'

"Sure, it'll sail on, but a lot of us will slip off the deck and drown."

I told him that since he was feeling better and had those eighteen hours of dialysis back in his life, he should go kick some butt. He laughed. "I promise I will," he said, "just as soon as I'm up to twenty ply."

I JOGGED LONGER and harder than usual while waiting to go back to Memorial, and drank much more red wine. When I felt the fist of anxiety in my chest, I concentrated on blotting out all thought with the yoga breathing exercises. If I get through this, I promised, I will pay back Shiva by learning to stand on my head.

I was nauseated the morning I went back—the classic reaction conditioned by those earlier chemo years—but I sensed almost immediately that the news was good. The nurse told me not to bother undressing, and the junior urologist came in without his senior, who was obviously no longer interested in my case. They had decided that the lump was just a variocele, part of a varicose vein, and no further treatment was indicated. Junior told me he'd thought a CT scan would be a good idea, but Dr. Wishy-washy hadn't thought it necessary, although both had agreed that with my history I should drop by Memorial every six months or so.

I broke out of the joint. I'm okay, I'm still a man. First thing, cut down on that red wine, big fella. And I'd probably break my neck trying to stand on my head, so let's scratch that. It's just a fucking varicose vein! No book, but that's cheap at the price.

It was almost a year before I found out the doctors were wrong, but it was a very good year.

7

SWEET, VAGUE Dr. Wishy-washy gave me no clue as he rolled my swollen left testicle between his fingers. This was ten months after I thought I was home free. Gasping, I asked, "So? If you were a betting man?"

He nodded, smiled at the wall, and softly said, "I would incline toward the benign."

It sounded like a song, "Incline Toward the Benign." But I didn't need a musical conductor right then, I needed a doctor to look me in the eye, outline the situation, help me make a decision, and then take on the problem. I needed a director for this sequel. I am the star, of course, but this is a big-budget, high-risk production and I can't do everything, especially since I'll be unconscious during some of the big scenes.

Dimly, I heard Dr. Wishy-washy say there are two options. One, we could wait several months, do yet another sonogram, and see if there is a change. Two, we could operate soon, and in the course of the operation take a biopsy; if the testicle is benign, we could return it to the sac, and if it is malignant, throw it away. If it is malignant, of course, there will be more tests, more treatments, and many more close encounters between us.

Which troubled me as I dressed and left. We did not have a long-term relationship, Dr. W. and I, and although I knew he was a respected urological surgeon, he did not give me that sense of confidence, that fighting edge I felt I needed. I was still comfortable with Memorial's no-nonsense, sometimes brusque approach. Whitmore and Chopp, Davor and Tom had always offered me straight talk along with hope. Now I was numb, except for my bowels, which were jittery.

Maybe I expected too much of Dr. W. Perhaps I was missing his signals. Was I wrong?

"You are right," boomed my friend Dr. Keith, a celebrated heart surgeon. "The patient-doctor relationship is critically important. Have I got a surgeon for you."

Dr. Burt, gruff and burly, saw me the next day, at another major-league hospital. With short-cropped hair and a G. Gordon Liddy mustache, he looked like a good candidate for medical editor of *Soldier of Fortune* magazine. I got the impression he could do the operation on his desktop with a Bowie knife using Jim Beam as his anesthesiologist. His sense of command was thrilling. I took notes as he told me we should get to it right away—with my history it was most likely malignant. He would remove the testicle, no biopsy, to avoid the risks of faulty pathology or spilling cancerous cells. He said all this with no tests and after an examination that barely ruffled my briefs.

"Just by looking into your eyes," he said, "I can see it's a teratoma."

I asked him about Dr. W.

"Competent," he said. When my raised eyebrows urged him on, he said that the operation was a simple one—a first-year urology resident could do it—but that I should be more concerned with the patient-doctor relationship. And then he asked, "Did you find him . . . wishy-washy?"

I was amazed that he used the phrase and I left exhilarated. I have found my Doc Director, I thought, the gung-ho, take-charge general/conductor/quarterback. But before I called his secretary to make the date, the exhilaration subsided and my stomach rumbled and the numbness settled into my shoulders.

Does it have to come to this, I thought, a choice between a doctor I can't read and one who wouldn't dream of letting me look at the script?

So I called Dave Kinne, the man I'd turned to thirteen years before, the man who'd operated on Margie ten years earlier. He reiterated how good a surgeon Dr. W. was, but allowed as how intangibles were important too. He gave me options. He would help me talk with Dr. W. or he could suggest several other urologists on the Memorial staff. I picked option two, and he picked Dr. Paul Russo, who, responding to Dave's call, saw me within hours.

Russo was thirty-eight, with the clean-cut, jut-jawed handsomeness of a comic-book hero. His crisp black hair looked almost Superman-blue. He seemed happy to see me, and although he churned along like a racewalker, he gave me full attention and did not seem to be rushing me out. He was clearly a product of the Whitmore-Chopp jock shop, brimming with self-confidence, the surgeon as athlete eager to get his hands on the ball, no pun intended. I all but swooned.

Of course, what he told me was not substantially different from what I had heard from Drs. Burt and W. The lump was definitely suspicious. We should get to it soon. After the initial operation, I could be out in a day or so. Even if the news was bad, the treatment was better now than it had been thirteen years before, and I'd made it this far, hadn't I? There was hormone replacement, testosterone.

We made a date, which he wrote down, pausing to explain that while he expected no problems, he would call to reconfirm after he spoke with Dr. W. It did not have to be said that he was younger than Dr. W. and inferior in rank. He said something about professional ethics. I barely heard that at first, for the numbness had gone, my stomach was quiet, and I felt easy for the first time in days.

And then later, angry, I thought: These doctors and their professional ethics; let's call it by its rightful name, office politics. We don't need socialized medicine as badly as we need more socialized people practicing medicine. That summer I had seen a movie, *The Doctor,* in which the hero, played by a handsome young William Hurt, gained humanity by getting throat cancer and finding out for the first time what his patients went through. He recovered to become a kinder, gentler doctor. It was not a good movie and it didn't quite ring true, although it was advertised as having been based on a true story. I eventually found that true story, a wonderful book called *A Taste of My Own Medicine* by Dr. Edward E. Rosenbaum. It was much grittier than the movie. Dr. Rosenbaum was in his seventies when his cancer was diagnosed, and when he finished his first trip through Malady as a traveler instead of a native he said, "I've switched sides. . . . If I could go back I would do things in my own practice very differently than I did."

As a patient, he knew too much. He saw potential errors in his diagnosis and treatment, and still was helpless. Worst of all for him was to be treated like a typical patient by rude clerks, patronizing residents, and attending doctors who made schedules for their own convenience and comfort, disregarding his pain and anxiety. He was concerned by doctors "becoming tradesmen . . . beholden to big business." Dr. Rosenbaum graciously concluded that "wisdom comes too late," so I felt a little mean-spirited wishing he had gotten his cancer forty years earlier, when it would have helped a generation of patients.

When Dr. Russo called back to reconfirm our date, he was almost apologetic about having had to talk with Dr. W. He didn't want me to think, he said, that he was "wishy-washy."

I managed not to laugh at those magic words, but couldn't resist saying, "Perhaps you should give me a local during the operation, so I can help you out."

"That won't be necessary," he replied with just enough starch to give me confidence. I told him to get his rest, eat well, do his finger exercises. It was his problem now. I liked it that he laughed.

WITH A WEEK to go before the operation, I determined to whip myself into the best physical shape possible. It was a week of eating well, of light drinking, daily yoga, and increasingly longer runs. The day before the operation, I decided to finish my training with a flourish, a five-mile run. In those days, three miles had been the absolute max. And thus I had my first—and so far only—mind/body experience.

My mind and my body have never been close. They coexist uneasily, one swaggering and overconfident, the other shy and self-conscious. My mind wishes my body was a more worthy container for such a hot property. My body wonders why my mind, if it's so smart, can't press the flesh into better shape.

My body occasionally complained about all the lard it had to lug, about huffing and puffing up gentle hills. Yet, for all those years on end, it never willingly skipped a single meal or passed up an extra buttered bagel, chocolate halvah bar, Hydrox cookie, spoonful of peanut butter.

I started out on the five-mile run through downtown Manhattan streets feeling good, but after two miles I realized it was going to be tough. So my mind, trying to help out or maybe just horn in, did something stupid. It bet my life. I told myself that if I made it all the way, if I ran the entire five miles, everything would turn out all right. The operation would be a success. The cancer would be curbed.

By the time I reached three miles, I understood the enormity of my mistake. I couldn't make it. No way. My breath was tangled in my ribs, my legs were rubbery, even my hair hurt.

Slow down, said my body. Stop.

But if you don't finish, said my mind, if we don't go the distance, we're history. We are dead.

My body ached and my mind felt fear, and for the first time in my life they got into sync. My mind and body were on the same page, they had merged into the same lane, they became . . . one.

I heard footsteps beside me and I sensed another runner. A voice said, "C'mon, whitey, you can do it."

It was Alfred Brooks, the skinny black high school dropout from *The Contender,* my first Young Adult novel. He was running beside me. I saw him.

"I made you up," I said.

"You made me up for this," he said.

I felt the presence of a runner on my other side.

"C'mon, fatty, pick it up." It was Bobby Marks from *One Fat Summer,* who lost all his weight pushing a lawnmower, just as I had.

"You can't run at all," I said.

"Maybe not in *your* book," he said.

And then came Jack Ryder, the high school baseball pitcher from *Jock and Jill,* and Sonny Bear, the half-Indian, half-white heavyweight boxer from *The Brave*—two big guys who ran ahead of me to clear the way, a good thing because my eyes were filled with water. I could barely see.

I ran the last mile blind. I don't know why I wasn't hit by a bus or a bike messenger, unless it was because Freddy Bauer, *The Chemo Kid* himself, hairless and swollen and tinged green, was up front stopping traffic and yelling, "C'mon, Lippy, you're the writer, you can pick any ending you want."

When I got home and collapsed, Kathy asked me why I was crying, and when I couldn't answer, she said, Don't worry, everything is going to be all right, and finally I said, I know everything is going to be all right, that's why I'm crying.

And then I told her this story, which is true. As I heard myself tell it then and as I read it now, I find it very hard to believe.

WHAT I REMEMBER best about the second orchiectomy was that the anesthesiologist, a woman I shall call Dr. Bea, said to me just before I went under, "Dr. Russo is terrific, he'll have your prostate out in no time."

When I started yelling, Dr. Bea scurried around until she found the computer mistake. She assured me that Dr. Russo would have caught the error on the table. (I have been assured that is true, but I also know that a brain surgeon at Memorial mixed up two patients with devastating results. Bad things can happen, and as long as you are awake it never hurts to check out whatever you can.) Dr. Bea continued telling the nurses about her recent vacation and I went to sleep to their oohs and aahs.

I woke up cold. Again. Hey, I wouldn't want Dr. Russo to have to sweat over me. And once again I woke up from an orchiectomy in a meat-locker room that looked like the set of a movie in which a doctor is storing bodies from which he will sell parts. Amazingly, once again, I awoke next to a very attractive young woman whose alluring shape was obvious under the sheets.

This time, I wondered if I would ever be aroused again.

I stayed only two nights in the hospital. It all happened so fast that I didn't even need to float a hernia story. As a matter of fact, I had never actually told either my parents— my mother had just been advised to have operations on both hands for carpal tunnel syndrome—or Kathy's widowed mother, slowly being crushed by osteoporosis. They both found out from *American Health* columns other people must have sent them. I sensed that they knew because of oblique questions that they asked, but none of them ever asked me outright. It seemed as though they were comfortable not dealing directly with the issue. I didn't think it was necessary to discuss the subject with them in depth since they were not involved as caregivers. Selfishly, I did not want to be answering interminable questions about my health, to be constantly frisked with their eyes at every family dinner. I did not want to be worrying about their worrying. On the other hand, if I had been in grave danger or terminal, I would have told them; elderly parents are concerned not only about their children but also about their dependence on their children, and they deserve to have information in time to make their own decisions.

Dr. Russo did not oooh and aaah over his scar. He said that there was not much more to do. There would be no retroperitoneal lymph node dissection—those nodes were long gone. He thought that there had been no spread, that the cancer had been caught early. We would keep a very close watch for a few years, he said, and if there were signs of spread, I would begin chemotherapy immediately.

The third night, near midnight, we began that very close watch with a CT scan in the dank bowels of the Memorial basement. The radiology machines down there seemed old and jerry-built—as it turned out, the department was moving to new quarters with more modern machines—and I felt part of a spooky experiment. When it was over, I was wheeled out into a dark corridor where Russo and Kathy were waiting.

"I'd really like to get out of here, right now," I said.

Russo let loose a cackle that reverberated off the dungeon walls. "Bug off, kids, I'll sign you out."

It felt like *The Great Escape, The Count of Monte Cristo, Papillon.* But I was a seasoned traveler now, and I knew better. The journeys to Malady are never over; they are over only for now. Celebrate everyday life.

A FEW WEEKS after the operation in the fall of 1991, I got my first shot of Depo-Testosterone, 200 mg. of a thick liquid injected into a muscle high on my buttock. It was designed to dissolve gradually into my system over the next four weeks, replacing the natural hormone from my missing testicles. If this would be the only price to pay for cancer, it would be a cheap one, I thought at first; no extensive surgery, no chemo, no radiation, not even a lot of fear and anguish.

But then I thought: I will have to have this shot, or some chemical implant yet to be devised, for the rest of my life. Without testosterone, I would risk hot flashes, osteoporosis, weight gain, and decreased muscle mass, not to mention the certain loss of libido and energy, and the possible alteration of my moods. With testosterone, there could be heavy sweating and bursts of short temper as side effects, and the terrifying future possibility that the testosterone would be creating a rapid river for the renegade cells of a prostate cancer. A common treatment for advanced prostate cancer is surgical or chemical castration.

And then there was the sense of dependency on a carefully controlled drug. My mother, among millions, gave herself daily insulin injections, and how many more millions took various critical medications. But still I found myself reading stories about cities under siege—Beirut, Belfast, Sarajevo—wondering what was happening to people cut off from their pharmacies. Were there men on testosterone unable to get their shots? What was happening to them? Loss of sexual function, low energy, what else? Was that loss reversible once you started getting your shots again?

Although I never kept a log of mood swings or sexual appetite, it seemed as though the shots gave me an even keel through the month; I might even be feeling more sexual and more aggressive than I had in recent months with one diseased testicle. I was quicker to stand my ground on the street. Once I chased a thief who had just plucked my dollar from a beggar's paper cup. Luckily, he got away. What would I have done with him? Twice, I got into physical fights, a pushing match with a bike messenger who sideswiped me while illegally riding on the sidewalk and a wrestling match with a cabdriver who illegally refused to pick me up, then grabbed me while I was writing down his number. Both men were bigger and younger than I, but my fury obviously scared them and they quit before I did. They thought I was crazy. So did Kathy and my kids, who were scared for me. I thought I was crazy too, but I sort of liked it. I also lashed out at people who I felt were being unnecessarily testy in conversation, to myself or others. I have consciously dialed down my temper, which leads me to believe I was allowing myself some bad behavior. But I still don't know if it was a psychological compensation for my surgical loss or a glimpse of the "'roid rage" that affects athletes bulking up on steroids.

There seemed to be little research on male hormone replacement. More than one of Russo's revolving Fellows asked me if I was able to have sex, and seemed surprised when I said there had been no diminishment of desire. The testosterone shots worked well, from the start.

By 1996, articles began appearing in medical journals with evidence that the athletes had been right all along; steroids absolutely increased strength and muscle mass. Soon, there were magazine stories about hormone *enhancement* for rich guys who wanted bigger muscles and more libido. This made me nervous; how would this affect price and supply?

For a fifties fatty who missed the Drug Culture, coming into the millennium with a monkey on my back seemed at first weird, even ironic. But then I thought, It's not as if you are mainlining heroin or sucking down reefers or snorting coke. You are doing anabolic steroids, such stuff as dreams are made on, the big-boy juice that makes heroes out of meatballs.

Such trash-think made me feel better immediately. After all, Arnold Schwarzenegger pumped himself up with steroids early in his competitive bodybuilding career, before such hormone use was controlled. He even admitted it on TV to Barbara Walters.

Of course, on 200 mg. a month I would never pump up, much less wipe out a bar with my bare hands just because the jukebox didn't have our song. I told Dr. Russo that if he would mega-jack my dosage, I could at least start competing in senior weightlifting events. I'd take him along with me to the next Olympics. He gave me his friendly cackle at that, and moved off to take care of sick people.

After more than five years on 200 mg., I took a test to measure the level of testosterone in my blood just before a monthly shot. It was extremely low. Russo later told me he ordered the test after hearing that another doctor's patient (I was Russo's only patient on replacement hormone therapy) was getting 600 mg. a month. My dosage was raised to 400 mg. and almost immediately I felt I had more energy, was more easily aroused sexually, and needed less sleep. It was not dramatic, but I did feel . . . better. Not that I had felt bad before, but I had been dragging a bit, which I had ascribed to pushing sixty while writing this book and two columns a week for the *Times*.

When I asked Russo and his nurse/assistant Susan Alfano why it had taken so long to raise the dosage, they explained that starting with a low dosage and working up is routine when there is no clear-cut formula. They reminded me that they were always asking if I felt tired or was having sexual problems, and I had always responded that I felt fine, which was true. I just could have felt better.

I'm still not sure about the lesson here, other than the old basic one: ultimately, we are our own healers. We have to listen to our bodies, we can take nothing for granted. These days, I keep hounding Russo and Alfano to raise my dosage again. Who knows how good I could feel. Wouldn't they like to go to the Senior Olympics as my trainers? They laugh and move on.

Not everyone found my dope dreams so amusing. One expert, Dr. Gary Wadler, who wrote a major text on the use of drugs in sports, has warned about a backlash. He has said that athletes, often with the complicity of coaches and athletic federations, are not only corrupting their sports and endangering their lives, but also giving bad names to good drugs that will become less accessible for real medical purposes. Like mine.

This was already happening. Testosterone is not readily available at my neighborhood pharmacies, and because most pharmacies—including Memorial's—would sell me only one month's dosage at a time, it was far more expensive than it need be. This had to do with laws passed to curb abuse by athletes and bodybuilders, who also helped give the hormone a bad name with a pattern of bar fights, gang rapes, and domestic abuse. There's a reason why so many women refer to macho posturing as "testosterone poisoning."

Had I been more sophisticated in the sixties when I went into National Football League locker rooms to interview those huge linemen with their coarse, pimply skin, thinning hair, cranky dispositions, and a constant yen for rough sex— all symptoms of steroid abuse—I would have known how important drugs had become in sports.

I covered the 1968 Olympics unaware that a dramatic sports revolution was emerging from the tip of a needle. Track and field athletes were suddenly bigger, stronger, faster, and they were recovering more quickly from minor injuries, which meant they could work out harder and more often.

Americans were scrambling for the drugs, then available without prescription, while many Eastern Europeans were getting them through official channels.

As steroid use became widespread among elite athletes, doctors, bureaucrats, and journalists variously denied its extent and efficacy or claimed it would cause instant death. While steroids can have disastrous and sudden side effects, thousands have used them to fulfill the Olympic motto (Higher, Faster, Farther), or just get better beach bodies through chemistry. Male gold-medal winners of my acquaintance, now in their healthy sixties, tell me how they carefully used the juice in precompetition "cycles," and female champions, who quit because of facial-hair growth and bone changes, talk nostalgically of the days when their strength and sex drive were racehorses they could barely keep in check.

Had these stories been as widely disseminated as the scare stories, had the pervasive use of steroids been understood, there might have been an intelligent examination of our brawling sports culture, and a sane public policy that might have curtailed some of the estimated 250,000 to 500,000 high school athletes who now dabble in steroids. Unfortunately, a kind of "reefer madness" about steroids developed, and young athletes, who believe they are immortal anyway, disregarded all the warnings because so many of them were bogus.

I still worry sometimes about my supply being cut off. Would I have to go to the black market, paying even more with less assurance the drug was clean, and become a criminal in the process? I felt a lot better when I found a pharmacy that would sell me a year's worth of shots at a time.

A FRIEND OF MINE, Dr. George A. Sheehan, the so-called "Running Doc" who found philosophical enlightenment in the marathon, took the drug GnRH to block his body's production of testosterone. It was an attempt to slow the spread of his prostate cancer. He chose chemical castration over the finality of a double orchiectomy. We began our relationship as writer and subject in the 1960s, later became fellow writers, then cancer buddies. We talked openly and at length. An erudite and witty man, George enjoyed telling me how much better, clearer, his mind was now that he wasn't being poisoned by testosterone. The Big T, he would say, stands for trouble.

"I am the eye in the sky now," he would say, "and I see how ludicrous men are, acting out a script written by a gland in their bodies. It's all testosterone. The only thing that protects us against it is good manners."

But that was the philosopher talking, not the jock. George was competitive, even if he was competing against his only truly worthy adversary, himself. How else explain his fierce will to win races, to better his personal bests, to set records into his seventies?

The reduction in testosterone may have been holding back the cancer, but it was also holding back George. It was slowing him down. He needed the natural juice to run fast. So he fiddled with the dosage in the daily GnRH injections, sometimes skipping them altogether when a race was coming up. He was willing to whittle days off the end of his life so he could be at his best. George made his death his own, as he had made his life his own, the object of research, metaphor, and tinkering. He *flirted* with death, which finally snatched him off the track four days before his seventy-fifth birthday.

We talked often during his final months in 1993, as I was coming up on the two-year anniversary of the second orchiectomy. I told him that Dr. Russo was very optimistic. The numbers and the CT scans were looking good, the monthly examinations were becoming more perfunctory. Russo saw two years as a significant mark. After that, the statistical likelihood of recurrence dropped sharply. But stats did not pacify me. After all, I had gotten this rare thing *twice*.

George could pacify me without lecturing me, just by offering himself as a brave and active model. Here I was whining about something that hadn't happened while he was trying to outrun Mr. Death. George wanted to finish another book, this one about his dying, called *Going the Distance*. He did, and it was published in 1996.

I miss George. He knew how to put life in perspective.

"I have come to believe," he told me once with a hint of edge, "that you shouldn't write about the marathon unless you've run it and you shouldn't write about cancer unless you've got it. And you shouldn't write about death unless you're dying."

8

ON FEBRUARY 8, 1995, I received an impersonal, fill-in-the-names-and-numbers form letter from a collection agency informing me that Memorial Sloan-Kettering's Outpatient Department had "referred" my account. I had five days to cough up $4,400.20. My first reaction, of course, was tumor humor. *So, what are you going to do if I don't pay, put back my cancer?* Then I felt a little sick. *Hey, leave me alone, I'm trying to find the cure for cash.*

With a headache and a stomach ache, both obviously cancer-related, I spent chunks of the next several days going through more than four years of bills, insurance claim forms, and canceled checks. I made a few phone calls, too. It didn't take long to figure out that it was my fault. I had lost control of my billing; I actually did owe them the money. The bottom line was that I would have to pay. The worst part was that if I had paid attention all along, I wouldn't have owed as much.

I began to wonder what it must be like dealing with such bills when you are really sick, alone, and unable to pay. Try to be funny about that, much less get a grip on it.

For reasons I don't completely understand, it wasn't until doctors began to complain that managed care was lowering their standard of living that the costs of trips to Malady became a serious subject fit to print. Even then, smart shoppers who routinely haggled with department store clerks and airline ticket sellers (and often got discounts) wouldn't dream of asking a doctor's fee up front. And it is only recently that people have begun to feel comfortable discussing their medical bills. I don't know whether it was a taboo or just considered poor manners, or, because insurance routinely paid, they didn't really know how much was being billed in their names.

I have been at dinner tables where men have casually recounted the side effects of their radical prostatectomies and women have bared their mastectomy scars, but none of them volunteered to talk about how much the operations cost.

Meanwhile, I still remember vividly the fortieth birthday party of a friend. His medical partners gave him a gold money clip inscribed with the date on which he broke their professional corporation's record for single-day billing. Most of the other party guests were doctors and their wives, and my friend got a standing ovation.

Money has always been a charged issue in Malady. Psychiatrists found a way to make the currency exchange part of the treatment, as if patients were shedding neuroses as they emptied their wallets. Other doctors pretended to be above the billing fray—until you couldn't pay. Stories of doctors who let bills slide for years or traded office visits in rural communities for farm produce or auto repair were rare enough to be worth Sunday supplement features.

Doctors have always worked pro bono, but that often included the required teaching and clinic appearances in return for affiliation at prestigious hospitals. In the early days of my medical travels, doctors could depend on an upper-middle-class life with very little bureaucratic oversight. Abuses of the system were so routine that they were considered part of medicine. Cost be damned, we've got lives to save, cried the doctors. And lives *were* saved. There were also unnecessary operations, profligate spending, duplicated machinery. For a while, doctors and hospitals grew rich. Insurance paid. If you had insurance. And even then, only up to a point.

The nightmare stories of people financially destroyed by illness, saddled for the rest of their lives with doctor and hospital bills, are too common for the Sunday feature spread. When I lived in a small suburban town, there always seemed to be a can alongside the local cash registers soliciting small change to help defray some neighbor's child's $250,000 bone-marrow transplant.

But sometimes I wonder whether big-ticket experimental procedures had less to do with the wreckage of the system than plain old day-to-day cash drawer greediness, a few dollars at a time.

A small example. Several years ago, an elderly woman I know became concerned about a number of annoying growths on her eyelids, tiny tags of flesh. She asked her ophthalmologist about them during a regular check-up. He said that he had noticed them, and that they should probably be snipped off before they grew larger. He could do it easily, he said.

"Why didn't you mention that before?" she asked.

"Because," he said, with a righteousness that pleased her, "I didn't want you to think I was drumming up business."

He made an appointment for the following week, in the hospital, so equipment and a nurse would be available. As it turned out, he needed no technology or extra hands, although he ended up spending an hour snipping off twenty-two tags.

Sometime later, he good-naturedly told the woman that he had a "confession" to make. Just as he was preparing to send Medicare a $400 bill for the "operation," he was informed that he'd be getting a check for $2,200.

"That's terrific," she said. "Then you won't mind paying the two-hundred-dollar bill I got from the hospital for the operating room we didn't use."

He recoiled, then decided she was being witty. She never did pay the hospital bill, and when the dunning letters stopped she wondered if he had paid it after all. She likes him, and so she never brought it up, and she didn't want her name used here because she intends to go back to him. But the story, which she frequently retells, still annoys her, not because it's a medical horror story, which it is obviously not, but because it's an everyday occurrence that is both cause and symptom of a system that needs treatment. Ultimately, who is supporting Medicare but working people, as she and her husband were and as her children and her grandchildren are? She has a similar story about a rheumatologist. She's afraid if she makes any complaints he will stop treating her.

In Malady, as we have come to accept, money represents comfort, proper care, dignity, and, too often, survival. There are deluxe tours and economy-class trips. The statistics about who lives and dies from similar diseases in Harlem and on Park Avenue may be chilling but they are not surprising. No wonder that those medical bills are inlaid with their own special dreads and angers: Will I have enough to get me to the end of treatment? Will I be working to support the doctors? Will I be making professional and personal choices based on keeping health insurance policies? Will I suffer or die because I can't afford top-of-the-line care?

The conventional wisdom seems to blame bureaucrats, politicians, insurance executives, Wall Street traders and corporate raiders for the increase in health-care costs (and they do deserve plenty of blame), but it has always been the doctors—the fee-for-service doctors, the incorporating doctors and the doctors whose wives jealously tend their books, the high-flying cosmetic surgeons, and the well-paid professors of medicine—who drove the engines of medical commerce. No matter how they postured as artists or scientists or saints, and many were all three, they all wanted to be paid, whether it was to finance their life-saving experiments or their second homes. They all claimed that since no price could be placed on health no one should be looking over their shoulders and marking price tags, like supermarket clerks. It was all between the doctor and the patient, they said.

Think of Dr. Burt's bill of $300 for a five-minute, second-opinion office visit in which he touched me lightly, glanced at the blood-test results and sonogram I had brought along, looked into my eyes and intoned, "Teratoma." When my eyes narrowed, he said: "I'm wrong about one in a hundred times, and I don't care."

His diagnosis turned out to be less than precise. In any case, my insurance company diagnosed his bill "in excess of customary and reasonable charges" and would pay him only $160 (80 percent of the $200 it decided the visit should have cost). I sent Dr. Burt's billing service $40 with a note asking him to explain why he was so excessive. No matter how unsatisfactory, I will pay the remaining $100 when that explanation arrives; that seems to be the way the system works. In my dread and desperation, I never asked him his fee up front. But I would like to hear what he has to say. We simply don't press doctors hard enough. Why are we so shy about money with them? Are we superstitious, afraid they won't like us enough to save us? Or is it that we are just too vulnerable, too scared, too distracted while we are trying to survive?

Ultimately, I am afraid that this issue may be completely taken out of our hands as the medical industry shakes out and cobbles together a managed-care system that works primarily in its own best interests. We need a Patients Union, something between the serious and useful approach of Consumers Union and the muscular intimidation of the Teamsters Union in their Jimmy Hoffa heyday, that will rate doctors and medical facilities, provide a decent price structure, and then throw up a line of beefy pickets if we're gouged or treated badly. Until that fantasy comes true, we'll have to muddle along, asking prices up front, disputing them later, when and if we can.

After more than five years, Dr. Burt has still never answered, even though I have gotten a bill for $100 from him or his various collection agencies regularly since, as well as numerous requests to send donations to his research projects. Once I got an invitation to attend a testimonial dinner in his honor at several hundred dollars a plate. I wish I could be precise about the amount, but I tore up the letter immediately.

Because my second major trip to Malady was pretty smooth as such trips go, I was able to focus on the exchange rate. I was treated well when it was important. Maybe I've been lucky so far because the nurses and technicians and support staff sang out, "Good luck," in their Las Vegas change clerk voices every time I went off to pull on a treatment slot machine.

I would, however, like to impose a "pain discount," especially from those phlebotomists who don't believe me that my big inner-elbow veins are dead from ancient chemo and insist on weaving in their needles, wiggling and grunting and getting angry when blood doesn't sluice out. After a while, they pull out, grin sheepishly, and go for the back of my left hand, which I have been waving in their faces.

"Should have listened to you," they chuckle, and when I say, "So how about a twenty percent rebate on your fee for the unnecessary suffering?" they chuckle louder and, I imagine, file the anecdote for those "krock" contests in which medics share stories about the cranky, ungrateful old patients who have not properly sucked up to them.

I would also ban "bill shuffling," in which, say, the cardiology department I've inadvertently overpaid because it billed both me and the insurance company sends the excess over to, say, the imaging department, which I've held off paying because its bill is wrong. Health-care providers seem to provide for each other first.

And I wish they wouldn't give out my name so easily. I

was hardly back home from the hospital before all the cancer organizations were asking for donations.

But how can I complain? It was a small cancer, after all, only about the size of a peanut, and although the medical-industrial complex billed $14,821.59 in its name for those three days and two nights in the hospital, I had to pay only $1,795.80 of it. Of course, all this was without a single blast of chemotherapy or radiation.

The largest single bill came from the hospital, $7,352.60, of which I had to pay only $11, for my telephone. Semi-private room rent for two nights was $1,870; surgery service was $2,560; the recovery room was $560, and that CT scan in the basement was $1,150 (later, I got one far more comfortably for $950 from an outside radiologist who suddenly raised his fee to $1,550 after "checking around" and finding his prices "low," then just as abruptly dropped it again after losing business). The rest of the bill was various tests and supplies.

Dr. Russo charged $2,000 to remove my diseased left testicle and drop in its place a silicone ball while I slept under the supervision of Dr. Bea, the anesthesiologist, who charged $1,105.

The union whose health insurance plan paid 80 percent of those charges, the American Federation of Television and Radio Artists, had recently invited Senator Edward Kennedy to speak on "Health Care: America's Sick Joke" at its convention. Senator Kennedy recounted some of his family's medical history, including his sister's retardation, one son's asthma, and another's bone cancer, which at one time cost $2,300 a month for chemo. Because the prosthesis his son wore in place of a leg had hinges, it was not covered. The Kennedys can afford any treatment. Many of them also have excellent coverage through corporations and government. I wish there were more senators on the case.

I would go on to have two years of monthly checkups ($75 for the doctor, $107 for the chest X-ray, and $206 for the blood work) and a CT scan every other month, a minimum of $20,712, of which I would pay something more than $4,000.

Just how much more I began to discover on January 26, 1994, when I called an account representative at Memorial because my bill, which for more than a year routinely showed several hundred dollars in credits (I was paying my bill before insurance was reimbursing the hospital) suddenly showed I owed $164 and included the footnote that I was "past due."

A rep named Barbara told me not to worry because the hospital was dealing with Blue Cross, which owed them nearly $4,000. When I kept asking her if I shouldn't do something, she got a little snippy and said, "Wait until we bill your insurance; I said it three times."

A month later, when my bill showed I owed $1,719 and was now "seriously past due," I called again. A rep named John said it was all "clerical," and there was nothing for me to do.

Like a dope, I did nothing, except marvel at the bills as they came in. There was a month I owed more than $6,000. ("Since you have failed to resolve your account in total, you leave us no alternative but to assign your account to our collection attorneys. Unless we receive payment within 10 business days, the process may commence.") But how could I take it seriously, when the next month the total would drop a few thousand without my doing anything? Numbers would shift from column to column on the bill from "Insurance Amount Billed" to "Patient Responsibility" and back again.

I didn't keep as careful a record as I had in the past because new tax laws denied deductions for unreimbursed medical expenses until they exceeded 7.5 percent of a taxpayer's adjusted gross income. Luckily, my expenses weren't that high. I figured if anything important happened, I'd get a call or a personal letter from Memorial. It never happened, and why should it? As I found out, many hospitals are not going to knock themselves out getting money from the insurance companies when they know they can sic collectors on us. While managed care may have begun as a good idea—to rein in doctors who were greedily feeding at the trough of insurance companies and tax money—it was quickly subverted into a way of speeding up the medical assembly line so profits could rise without necessarily raising fees.

On February 9, 1995, just a little over a year from my chat with Barbara and one day after I received that printed form from the collection agency, I called Memorial again and got Barbara again.

No point coming in to work this out, she told me cheerfully, it's too late; it's between you and the collection agency now. She hung up.

The collection agency sent me several more printed forms, then a printed letter ("It is difficult for us to understand why you have chosen to ignore . . .").

One day there was a message on the answering machine from someone named "Woody" who said he was calling from a lawyer's office. Eventually there was a printed form letter from the lawyer ("This office has been engaged to proceed against you . . ."). By that time I had finally sat down and done the painstaking paperwork I should have been doing all along. Memorial may well have been right that it was owed that money (there are, by the way, private firms who will audit your health bills for a fee). But some of the responses Memorial got from several insurance carriers about what they did or did not cover should have been challenged, as should have some of the bills that Memorial sent to the insurance company. Memorial did not follow up the way I would have if I had been taking care of business. And by not challenging Memorial's bills, I had blown deadlines.

A rep named Romeo at Memorial was helpful and explained how "the system generates numbers" from column to column on the bill based on how much time has gone by and not on whether or not money has actually changed hands. The hospital, he said, bills the insurance carrier as "a courtesy" to the patient and rarely makes more than one pass at collection unless more than $500 is involved.

So I paid the bill and began digging out individual charges I might still be able to challenge. In one case, insurance had rejected a $799 charge that they should have paid because Memorial submitted it more than 15 months after the service, past the time the insurance company considered claims. I tried but was unable to resurrect that one. There were others.

A few weeks later, I got a new bill from Memorial for $319 ("Since you have failed to resolve . . ."). I called the insurance company and found out they had already responded to that claim with a check to Memorial for $239.25. I sent Memorial $79.75 to make up the difference, the patient's responsibility. I marked it all down on my new chart. A tiny victory in my new campaign.

I felt pretty stupid about all this, but since then I have been on the case. Line by line. And I have come to realize that the bottom line is this: Getting reimbursed, like getting well, is basically the patient's responsibility.

If you're well enough to do it, that is.

Of course, if some tiny renegade cell is roaming your system and decides to set up shop in lung or brain, if your arteries jam or your immune system declares bankruptcy, you could be looking at six figures real fast, enough to break some professional corporation's gross record if it doesn't break you first. It is important that you or someone you trust keep a running log of medical visits, what was done and what was charged, paid, reimbursed. Keep a list of your follow-up calls, with the name and number of the person with whom you spoke. Keep a calendar of the deadlines for filing claims and for challenging medical charges and insurance reimbursement decisions.

But nothing is as important to the process as an hour or two of prevention, the paperwork version of the routine checkup. Read your health insurance contract. It is a chore we all want to ignore or delay, but you have to do it, and you have to do it when you are alert. Make notes on the margins of the policy, be satisfied that you know exactly what is covered and what isn't, that this is the coverage best suited to your needs. Don't be shy about calling up for more information. They won't be shy about calling up for more money.

9

MY DAD AND I wait at the border of Malady, a country in which he has never traveled, although he is ninety years old. We tensely sit in molded red plastic chairs in the narrow hallway that connects the doctors' offices in a big old wooden house in a small upstate New York town. We are waiting for one of the doctors to call us in and discuss what he's learned from the X-rays of my father's gastrointestinal tract. I think that both of us are scared, although I'm only sure that I am. Dad has always kept his feelings private. But I know how important control is to him, and once he crosses that border into the country of illness, the simplest aspects of his life will be out of his hands.

My dad has never before admitted to being sick. He was born at home in 1904, and he was a hospital patient only once, in 1956, when he had a hernia repaired. He had an allergic reaction to penicillin that reinforced his distrust of doctors. He is about 5 feet 5 inches tall now, shrunk from about 5 feet 7 inches, medium for his time. People find him "cute." He has a white mustache and goatee, which gives him the look of a retired professor, and the chunky, muscular body of a retired construction worker. He has always enjoyed sounding erudite while bustling around like a handyman. This past winter he shoveled the snow off his driveway and this summer he tilled his garden and planted tomatoes. He can sit very still, reading, for hours, then jump up and buzz around the house doing chores, trot down to his basement library, climb up on the roof to fix a flapping shingle. He was a track athlete in high school—I found that out by discovering some old medals in the back of a drawer—but he never participated in sports in my lifetime. He started each morning with his "calisthenics" in the shower, a flurry of arm-waving and grunting. Then he emerged to charge into his day.

But now, for the first time in my memory, he looks, as my mother described him over the phone the night before, like "a crushed old man." He has been weak, nauseated, running a fever, unable to eat for several days. Over the years he has occasionally been, as he would say, "under the weather" or "fighting a cold," but he would slink off into a corner with a book and a cup of tea until he felt better, like an animal crawling into a cave. He might even growl at my mother if she tried to minister to him, or asked him too often how he felt.

But he must think something is really wrong this time because he is allowing us to help him. And he is depending on me to be his guide and interpreter in the country of illness. I hope I am up to the job. For all my scars and attitude, I wonder if I really know enough about the place to help him.

Rain rattles the skylight above us and a heavy young woman in white—receptionist, clerk, technician?—cries out, "Oh, my tomatoes are saying, 'Thank you, Lord, thank you.' " She looks around for audience reaction.

Dad does not react. He doesn't yet know about sucking up to the border guards, the petty bureaucrats, the gatekeepers of Malady. He has no idea how important they are, how they can ignore you to death.

This old Malady hand smiles brightly at the heavy young woman in white. I would applaud her little performance to get my dad better service. Call it Uncle Tomming, call it flirting, call it finesse; it's about survival. Another old patient sitting in our row of plastic chairs engages her in a discussion of gardening techniques. Smart. It could get a quicker appointment next time.

I want to nudge my dad, urge him to get in on this conversation, to make himself human to the gatekeeper with a description of the small, green tomatoes he left home alone. But it's too early in the trip to push him so hard and maybe, if we're luckier than I feel, it will be unnecessary; the rest of the journey will be canceled.

But I sense we are committed to the trip. Six days ago, after he felt shooting pains in his stomach, Dad began dosing himself with Tylenol, a major event. He does not believe in drugs of any kind, much less alcohol or more than one cup of caffeinated coffee a day. He has never smoked. He has always been physically active. He believes in moderation, the only one in the family who does, and is always declaiming at mealtime, "Jefferson said you should always leave the table a little hungry."

When I was younger and sassier, I would snap back, "And Ben Franklin said you should finish anything that Jefferson left." A tolerant man, Dad laughed the first hundred times or so.

My mother is eighty-six. She is worried that Dad might have caught a virus—in the summer of 1994, the flesh-eating virus was in the news—and she was afraid that he would die overnight. Dad thought it might have been a pepperoni sandwich and he was worried that the lunch meats he loved were finally getting to him.

I heard all this by phone on a Sunday evening. By the time I drove up to see him on Monday morning, he was sitting in a corner of the enclosed porch, his favorite room, reading, sipping tea, being cranky. What alarmed me were his unshaven cheeks. Here was a man who shaved every single day, even if his only appointment was with green tomatoes.

"So how do you feel?"

"Better." He held up the book he was reading. I thought it was typical of him to put a book up between himself and reality. "I think you should read Trollope again. There's more to him than you think."

"I never read him in the first place."

He sighed. "An ignoramus for a son. While you're up here, we'll get some books for you to read."

My mother rolled her eyes. "He's been an impossible patient."

"He's been lucky," I said. "He doesn't know how to be sick."

My mother's most regular doctor—she has a staff because she has never been regularly well—was on vacation. My parents didn't want to go to a doctor who didn't know them, who would see only two old people, not the active, thinking, passionate editors of their quarterly temple bulletin, vibrant co-conspirators of life.

I pressed them to think of a doctor, any doctor, perhaps someone they knew socially, more likely the middle-aged son of someone they knew socially. I'll call him up, I said, describe the emergency, and ask for a quick referral to an internist.

When they recoiled from asking for a favor—or could it be from admitting a lack of control?—I explained that this was no favor, that hero docs liked nothing better than to shoot their cuffs and come up with an easy solution to a simple problem that costs them no time or money.

My parents found this a little cynical, but they liked my tough-guy take-charge approach and trusted me enough to rummage through their address books and come up with a name. The doctor seemed delighted by my call. Within fifteen minutes, he called back with not only the name of an internist "your pop will love, a character just like him," but also a confirmed appointment in one hour.

My parents thought I was a genius, which I loved, even

though I really felt like one of those sly fixers you hire in Eastern Europe, Central America, the South Bronx, to drive, change money, interpret, keep you from getting ripped off by anyone except their friends. You need fixers in Malady too.

But even with the metaphor in place, I recalled how for many years my father refused to travel unless he could drive to the destination. I had assumed back then he would never give up control to an airline pilot, to lose the power to turn off the road or turn around. And then, sometime in his late six-ties, my parents flew to Europe on a group charter, survived and became frequent fliers for a few years. Which meant they could change their ways if they wanted to or had to.

We drove to the referred doctor's office, the old house two towns away. My parents were complimentary about my driv-ing and my sense of direction, neither of which is notable. I sensed a shifting of responsibility. It was too early to feel un-easy, but I remembered the weekly trips to my mother's hand surgeon the previous year. She had carpal tunnel surgery on both hands, performed by a friend's son in New York City. Every visit required me to make two 3½-hour, city-country-city round trips in a day, and toward the end I was driving too fast—eventually 75 miles an hour in a 35-mile-an-hour Thruway construction zone, which required some lawyering from another of their friends. The fault was totally mine; nei-ther of them was telling me to drive faster, but I later came to realize that what was making me so nuts was my dad's denial.

He totally zoned out during those trips, reading, chatter-ing about national politics, pretending it was a kind of out-ing, a family day trip. While he was very attentive to my mom, and more than willing to take over the shopping, cooking, and cleaning while she recuperated, he simply would not become engaged in the medical aspects. He would stay in the doctor's outer waiting room while I went inside with Mom and he would never join the medical discussions afterward. He would interject something he had just read in *Time* magazine about foreign policy. He did not want her sick. He refused to cross the border with us.

But when we get to the doctor's office this time, it is my mom who stays out in the waiting room. I go in with my notebook open and take ostentatious notes while my dad's pale, chunky, amazingly fit body is thumped and prodded and X-rayed. It may have been the first time he has ever been X-rayed by a private doctor, the first time, except for the hernia, that he underwent an examination that was not part of his employment physicals.

The doctor seems slightly put off that there is not much medical history before this week. "When did you have your last exam?"

"Before you were born," says my father.

"I doubt that," snorts the doctor. Other than being a little loud and smug, I don't think he is such a character.

"It was before my last promotion at the Board of Education in New York," says Dad. I am amazed at how smoothly he slips in some biography. Is he consciously working the doctor, setting up class bonds, humanizing himself? "That would be 1959."

"I was twelve years old." The doctor looks faintly interested now.

"Aren't you going to ask me my age?"

"I'll get to that."

"It might be part of the prognosis." The professor is emerging.

The doctor's sigh is comic. "Okay, how old are you?"

"You guess."

"Seventy-four."

"You are a gracious gentleman. I am ninety."

I think the doctor is surprised, although he tries to look as though he really knew all along. I am impressed at how my father is sliding into all this. But, of course, you don't get to be ninety without some moves.

"Let's look at the pictures," says the doctor, pointing up at the X-rays clipped to a light screen on a wall. He points out what he describes as a blockage in the colon and a white badge that he calls a calcification.

One of his partners swaggers into the room, glances at the X-rays, and announces that it is a gallbladder attack. They argue in doc dialect, but both agree that Dad should go to the hospital right away.

Dad does not want to go. He says he is already feeling better.

The doctor says to me, as if Dad isn't there, "If this was my grandfather, I would make him go. I would not take no for an answer."

We are ushered back out into the hall to make our decision. Do we make this border crossing? We sit down in the plastic chairs. Dad looks at me. "What do you think?"

"It's what do you think," I say.

"I think doctors make you sicker. I don't think they know what they're talking about. They can't even agree on what they think is wrong. If I go home and rest, I'll feel better in a few days."

"So why are you asking me?"

"You have a lot of experience in these matters," he says. There is no implication that I am wiser, merely unluckier. "You know more about doctors and hospitals than I do."

He is asking me to make the decision. It is not easy, I think. I know too much. But do I know enough? My father knows his body. It is very possible he is right, that it was the pepperoni, which will eventually work its mischievous way out of his system. But even so, the process may have left him so weakened and vulnerable that he needs hospital care to regain his strength.

I know that doctors and hospitals are not always reliable; there are medical mindsets as hidebound as religious dogma and there are economic agendas that can work against an individual patient's health. You can never be sure that the high-tech machine examining you isn't really a calculator. You can never be sure that someone touching you, be it chief of the service or linen-changer, has washed hands properly since touching someone with an infectious disease. But if Dad really needs medical attention, a hospital makes more sense than a corner of the porch.

For selfish reasons, I shrink from the responsibility. If he goes into the hospital, I will have to become an active watchdog. More important, how can I bear the guilt if my advice sends him home and I am wrong?

Finally, I say, "If you go in, they will put you on the medical conveyor belt, poke and prod you, give you tests, maybe make you sicker in the short run. It could be a waste of time and money."

He is nodding, but listening carefully. I pick my words and lean close to him. I don't want to shout, but I want to be sure he hears each word.

"On the other hand, if there is something wrong, and you don't go in, you could die. Which is not an acceptable risk."

He thinks about that for a moment, then says, "Okay," in the same tone he used fifty years before when I begged him to take me swimming when he wanted to keep reading on the porch. "Tell your mother. Let's go."

I feel fear in my stomach. God, I hope I'm right. I hope I really do know enough about doctors and hospitals. I hope I got something out of all those trips to Malady.

I HAD ALWAYS thought of my father as a macho man. Not the obvious and ersatz macho—call it crotcho—of muscle-flexing, teeth-sucking, flashing the wad, but that contained macho of not complaining, not explaining, of never asking directions, of being willing to take charge and take responsibility. I had loved to visit him at his school when he was a principal. He said that being principal was the closest thing to being captain of a ship, and he certainly was a prideful, though benevolent, leader. Captain Kirk on the bridge of the starship *Enterprise*. The schools he ran were tough schools, in those days publicly labeled for the "emotionally disturbed and socially maladjusted," although the names were later changed to protect the kids from lifetime stigma.

I saw my father pull knives out of students' pockets, and now and then deliver a wallop to the seat of a big kid's pants. The kid invariably grinned, grateful for the contact, glad that someone cared enough. Dad had only hit me once that I remembered, an open-handed slap across the jaw that knocked me off my chair at the dining table. I had just said something too fresh to my mother.

Sitting at the borderline that day, I wasn't ready yet to be his father, but I had to be his advocate, his protector in the hospital. And, in my deepest fear, I might have to help him die. So what did I know? That's all I thought about after my mom and I checked Dad into the community hospital, had dinner, and I began what would be a daily commute from the city. The idea of Malady was born on the highway as I tried to answer that question. So what *did* I know? Not that much. At first, because I thought of Malady in the large geopolitical way in which Sunday morning TV talking heads discuss whole continents ("Africa must decide if it will align itself with Asia . . ."), I was overwhelmed by the size and complexity of "the health-care system," in which monolithic institutions staffed by professionals with mysterious knowledge and cryptic styles of communication made life-and-death decisions.

It took a while to break it down. There is no "system." If there was, there would be a central intelligence, an attempt at efficiency, cooperation, a vision. Instead, there is a wasteful, inefficient, sometimes chaotic scramble for financing, facilities, and customers, as in most other businesses. Predatory corporations are moving in to dam up rivers of cash. The hospitals are dedicated to their own survival. The doctors, even the best of them who originally signed on to save people, are caught between doing good and doing well. Too often that's a conflict, and it's becoming more of one.

That's all theory, and this has to be practical, I thought as I drove. Let's keep it simple. Focus on the doctor, more specifically the doctor's relationship with my father, as the surest way to get the best service. We'll need an accessible line of communication, and we'll have to keep up the pressure so the doctor will quickly diagnose the illness and cure it. Make sure the doctor is interested and active. This is the key. Most everything else is comfort and money. We also need to be alert against mistakes, and to be sure that choices are made in Dad's best interests, not because of his age or because of cost efficiency or because some specialist or nurse or X-ray reader wants to leave early for a kid's piano recital.

My own experience had been lucky. With an ambassador like Dave Kinne offering his letters of introduction, I had gotten to Whitmore and then Russo, each the right doctor for the time. Kinne himself had been the right one for Margie. But Dave had been a social friend and that had immediately made a difference. I had to find a way for Dad to crack through into the doctors' consciousness. Would I have to make a lot of noise, invoke experts from the city? Should I call my friend Mark, a major league gastroenterologist? Mark had played in my house as a kid; he knew Dad well.

But my parents felt strongly about staying in this local hospital, and going to the city might be more stress than it was worth. Could Mark consult with Dad's doctors, or would that alienate them? Maybe I could gather enough information so I could have Mark counsel me. How far could I intervene; how far would my parents let me? How much responsibility was I ready to take?

The dynamics of an elderly patient and a grown-up child are likely to complicate the Malady trip, and guilt is a certain side effect when things go wrong. The eighty-five-year-old mother of my friend Roy Nemerson had a clogged aortic valve that her doctors said needed to be replaced. (Arnold Schwarzenegger elected to have that heart operation at forty-nine, while he was still strong and young.) Ann Nemerson's heart bled uncontrollably during the operation and she died the next morning. Roy and his father remembered a doctor quoting a 10 percent mortality rate for the operation in a brief, unsatisfying pre-op discussion. Meanwhile, the medical records noted "a long, long review" with the family, and doctors later claimed a 50–50 risk. Was there an unseemly rush to operation? Did the surgeon, who first met Roy during a break in the operation, know all the facts in the case? Should he have stopped when he saw the bleeding? Did the operation cause the bleeding? If there was a failure of communication, who was it between and when did it happen? Roy has gone over the case a dozen times in his head, sent letters and called, in vain, for an investigation. He keeps wishing he had not trusted the doctors, that he had gotten a second opinion.

After I wrote about Roy and his mother, a number of people called and wrote with similar stories that were haunting them. Neal Rauch had made an appointment for his seventy-two-year-old mother to get a second opinion after doctors advised an operation with "only a 1 percent fatality rate" to repair an esophageal hernia that was causing frequent vomiting. Florence Rauch suffered from osteogenesis imperfecta, or congenital brittle-bone disease, which had eventually put her in a wheelchair. She was otherwise in good health. She refused to go for the second opinion because she just wanted to get the operation over with. It was a success, but she died the next day. A blood clot had gotten into her lung. Some time later, a cardiologist casually mentioned to Neal's father that Florence had been at much higher risk than average because she was sedentary. Neal still wonders, Didn't her surgeon know that? And, Was there something else I should have done?

In most such cases, there is plenty more we should have done and we probably would have done it if we hadn't been stymied by a lifetime of our parent–child relationship. Do the best you can, but don't beat yourself up over it. Remember that old line about parents, They can push all your buttons because they put them there. Just because they are old and sick and dependent on you, don't think you can easily take charge in Malady.

I hadn't figured all that out yet in the summer of 1994 when I sailed into Dad's hospital room filled with the resolve to meet whatever the challenge might be—and fighting off the dread of what I might actually encounter. Which turned out to be a jolly old dad sitting up in bed, looking good, busy discussing Freud with his roommate, who happened to be a counselor at a nearby juvenile facility, a blue-collar guy with a white-collar education, exactly the kind of person my father liked to hire as teachers.

The roommate was wearing a green golf shirt and shorts as he lounged in bed, as if it were a chaise by the pool. He was holding on to his own identity in this place.

Not Dad, who had slipped right into the program. Not only wasn't he wearing the pajamas and robe we'd brought for him, but he also seemed very comfortable in the frayed hospital gown, with his bottom hanging out. If the IV needle in his arm was bothering him, you didn't know it. He seemed to be wearing it.

Meanwhile, the doctors, who still didn't have a clue what was wrong, had begun ordering every test they could think of, in between dropping by to argue politics. Both of which were fine with Dad, he told me, because it broke up the day. There was only so long you could read, he said, before you wanted to get out and do something.

That night my car broke down and I waited hours for a tow truck. I looked much worse than Dad the next morning, which he noted. He demanded an explanation. He shook his finger at me and the IV stand wobbled.

"Don't ever underestimate the toll that car troubles take on you," he said. "The helpless feeling, the loss of independence and control. You wonder what's going to happen next."

"Shouldn't I be saying all this to you?" I asked.

"I've got no problems," he said, whipping the IV lines. "It's the doctors' problems."

As hospital stays go, his trip to Malady turned out to be a leisurely packaged bus tour. The doctors might not know what was wrong with him, but whatever it was, it was fading rapidly. The pains were gone, his energy was returning. Nothing beats a good rest and a liquid diet through the arm.

His next roommate was another jovial, salt-of-the-earth guy, a heart patient who introduced us to his family and told stories about his union. When he heard one day that it was my parents' sixty-first wedding anniversary, he ran out to get a card at the gift shop and alerted the nurses, who made a fuss.

The nurses, as they often are in community hospitals, were friendly and attentive, quick to notice a swelling in Dad's arm from the IV, and responsive to his deadpan humor.

I walked in one day while a nurse was giving him a sono-gram. As the wand came close to his still-distended belly, he asked, "Any signs of life in there?"

Without missing a beat, she said, "My goodness, I had no idea you were expecting."

"They didn't inform you I was a hermaphrodite?"

You'd have thought it was Comedy Central.

Dad had also managed to punch through to the doctors. His age and lack of medical history made him interesting. The fact that I came up from the city in tie and jacket, and was of their age and class, made them responsive to me as well. Unfortunately, their information was often conflicting and sometimes sounded highly speculative; there was much talk of secondary inflammations and reflex slowings of the system, all caused by primary events of which they didn't have a clue. They didn't know what to do. But doing nothing seemed to be making Dad better by the minute.

His third roommate was an old man (even Dad, probably ten years older, referred to him as an old man), obviously very sick and in great pain. He groaned constantly, spilled food, and soiled himself. The room stank, and it was hard for Dad to sleep. Mom and I wanted Dad out of the room, but Dad was sympathetic to his roommate. He thought the old man wasn't getting enough attention from the nurses, and he thought he should stay there so he could ring for a nurse when the old man was in trouble. The principal was taking charge again.

At that point, it seemed like the time to go home. The doctors were against discharging him—they were thinking up new tests—but I was insistent, and we made a deal: we would stay in close touch; if he felt nauseated or didn't have bowel movements, I'd bring him right back.

I am not much of a letter-writer, but I must have needed to start putting things down because I wrote to Susannah, who was traveling that summer in another dangerous and complicated place, Eastern Europe and Russia. I wrote:

Brought Grandpa home from the hospital a week ago, he was feeling much better but we were still in the dark as to what caused his illness. (Still are.) This all complicated by the turf wars of the docs—the gallstone-mason claimed his fever–weakness–nausea, etc., was caused by gallbladder attack which needed to be laser'd, while the gastronaut said it was from a partial blockage in the colon which needed to be opened. In any case, taking him home was risky—he needed to go from IV to solids and to pass waste through the nar-rowed colon or he would be back and sicker.

Well, he did his duty and he's feeling pretty good although he doesn't understand why after all that time in the hospital he doesn't feel like he did when he was, say, 70. He's tired. He'll go back for more checkups, and in a week or so the gastro guy will work a tube into his colon with a balloon attached, then blow up the balloon to attempt to make the opening in the colon larger.

It was kind of weird being his tour guide—it was not one of those classic reversals where I became the par-ent, etc., but more like the money-changer/fixer you probably could use; he depended on my knowing my way around Malady (you like that name?), when in fact all I really have is a bad attitude. But that seemed to be enough—Grandpa slipped into denial (he was there to read and chat with his roommates, whom he liked, and flirt with nurses) while Grandma was sur-prisingly docile with the docs. Gale and I still can't sort it all out.

More than three years later, my sister Gale and I were still trying to sort it out. It may well have been the pepperoni after all. The terrible irony, of course, was that soon after Dad came home from his little Malady getaway, Margie took off on the grand tour.

I O

IN THE SUMMER of 1994, Margie went to France on a group art tour. She loved the confluence of pleasures—travel, education, conversation, painting. But when the group spent a few days in a castle, she found herself huffing and puffing up and down the steep stone steps. Sometimes she had to push herself to keep up with the group. She attributed it to age—she was sixty-two—but many of her traveling companions were older. She felt numerous aches and pains, in particular a stabbing pain in her buttocks that ripped down her leg. She thought it was sciatica.

One night, in bed, trying to fall asleep in the recommended fetal position for lower-back problems, fantasizing about starting to paint again when she got home, she felt a "bullet" ripping into her coccyx. It left her breathless. Her first thought was, "This is it"; after thirteen years, her cancer had recurred.

Slowly, the pain subsided. Through the night, waiting for it to return, she imagined herself in the north light of her Manhattan apartment, mixing paints, handling brushes again. In 1963, when we began living together, she had just started selling her oils. She even had a one-person show at the *Times*. I made the frames for her paintings.

The bullet pain did not return that night, or ever again to that place. She decided she was wrong. If it was really cancer, she thought, the pain wouldn't have gone away. She began to forget about it.

Back in New York that fall, she reached into the dishwasher one morning and felt something snap in her right side. Later that day, a neighbor in the elevator noticed the mask of pain on her face, heard the story, and told her that a broken rib could puncture a lung and collapse it. Better see a doctor immediately.

Her regular doctor, an internist at Memorial, was on vacation, so Margie went to the Cancer Center's version of an emergency room, the Urgent Care department. She was put in bed and tests were taken. The covering doctor said that her blood count was low and offered a transfusion, which Margie rejected. As it turned out, she had a form of anemia that strikes cancer patients whose tumors are attacking the bone marrow.

When her doctor returned, Margie had a bone scan. She was well aware that when breast cancer recurs, it often appears first in the bones. She waited five days for the results. Why, she thought then, had her doctor not ordered bone scans before; at least there would be a baseline against which the new scan could be compared.

When the doctor called, she said: "I have bad news. The bone scan shows cancer. There's also good news. It's not in any organs."

Margie buried her head under the covers and cried. She also screamed out, "He won!"

She didn't tell me this until eighteen months later, in February 1996, on a day she was half out of her mind on morphine and Ativan. I sat stunned, in a corner room of the eighteenth floor of Memorial, staring out at the river. It was a big, sunny room, and she was in it alone because she had cried out in pain so often that her roommate asked to be moved in the middle of the night. I stared at the river, trying to tune in to the feelings she had brought up in me.

Was I feeling guilt that my cancer was lesser? Testicular, even the second time around, is rarely as dangerous as a metastatic recurrence of breast cancer. I must have sat there for a long time without talking because Margie said, "I shouldn't have told you; you're upset now."

I admitted that I was upset and that I was struggling to figure out exactly why. She told me not to be upset, that it had all grown out of a fight we had had a week before she got the diagnosis a year and a half earlier. Didn't I remember? I didn't, but then my memory had never been as deep and precise as hers. She said that we had had lunch at a deli on the Upper West Side to talk about the kids. Somehow it had slipped into sharp words about alimony. I said she was getting too much, she said too little, and we stalked apart. A week later, when she got the news of metastasis, her thought, "He won," meant that I wouldn't have to pay her alimony much longer.

Back home that night, I went through my calendars for 1994 and 1995, looking for the day that Margie and I had had the lunch and the quarrel over alimony. It was on October 5, 1995, a full year after she got the bad news. In her drugged state, she had collapsed time. There was a clear lesson in that; you can't quite trust what a person says while taking heavy painkillers. Listen through a filter.

Cancer brought us back together. We began to talk regularly on the phone, filling in pieces of our lives apart. She had been taking Prozac since we split in 1988, when her therapist said, "Do something nice for yourself." She had been feeling pretty good, she said, until November 1991, when she began to feel pain in her ribs and back, annoying but nothing like the pain she would feel three years later in France. In retrospect, it was probably the first signal of the cancer's spread.

Her internist did not suggest a bone scan in 1991, perhaps because she was so busy fending off Margie's insistence that the pain was due to her large left breast weighing her down and throwing her off-balance. When Margie suggested that the breast be removed, the doctor dismissed that as "radical," even though it had been an option back in 1981. I never understood how Margie was persuaded to have the breast reduced in size and to have reconstruction on the right side. She had always been disdainful of reconstruction. Had she turned herself over to her doctor too blindly? She had no trusted sidekick at that moment.

During the reduction, a few "microscopic isolated cancer cells" were found, she remembered being told, but no one seemed that concerned. Kinne suggested she think about entering a Tamoxifen study, but her doctor vetoed that, said Margie, warning that Tamoxifen could cause uterine cancer.

During this period she was also disturbed by the intermittent swelling of her right arm, a condition called lymphedema. Scar tissue from the 1981 mastectomy was blocking the drainage of lymph fluid. Dave Kinne had been very aware of the danger back then and urged Margie never to pick up heavy objects, like suitcases, with her right hand, and to take special precautions not to be cut or scratched or burned; she should always wear a glove in the kitchen or garden, and with pets. This is good advice, but hard to follow for an active woman who wants to have a normal life. But without lymph drainage, everyday infections could become dangerous; a simple cut that most people treat themselves would be worth a trip to Urgent Care.

These days, there seem to be more aggressive techniques, pumps and procedures to bring down the swelling before the skin of the arm loses its elasticity. A promising new technique in which only so-called "sentinel" nodes are removed and examined, thus avoiding the stripping out of many nodes, may save thousands of patients from lymphedema. Once the swelling begins, however, it is hard to get it back down. Margie tried elevating her arm, wearing a tight support glove, getting massages from a physical therapist, even renting an electrical pump, but the swelling was advanced.

In January 1992, she began the reconstruction process, which was more painful and time-consuming than she had imagined. The left breast was reduced in size, and an empty sack called an expander was sewn into her chest on the right side. Over the course of several months, the sack was enlarged with injections of saline, stretching out the skin. In April, the sack was removed and replaced with a permanent implant. Margie was never really happy with the look or feel of the reconstructed right breast. It had no nipple and never matched the reduced left breast.

She wondered if she had not researched the matter carefully enough, or had not been given enough information. We decided it was a combination of both, plus the doctors' routine assumption—their so-called quick reads—of what the patient wanted. As is so often the case, the doctors didn't take the time to find out what the patient really wanted and needed, and the patient had let things just happen, wanting to believe that the doctor really did know.

Margie often thought later that the "drastic" choice of removing the breast would have been the best, less painful and less expensive. Of course, the best choice might not have been a cosmetic choice at all but a medical choice, including those unordered scans, in which the metastasis would have been found sooner, and perhaps even stalled or beaten back for a while.

THE DAY MARGIE found out, I was one of the first two people she called with the news. The other was her cousin Betty Abeles. She felt that both our responses were entirely appropriate.

Betty said, "Oh, shit."

I said, "I'm so sorry."

Then she told a third person, a friend who began to tell her about someone she knew who had lived for many years with metastases of some other kind of cancer. Margie almost hung up on her, but then decided to give a lecture instead. Mindless cheerleading is no help, she said, and neither is crêpe-hanging. Nobody with any sense wants to be trivialized or patronized when the roof seems to be caving in. You want to be listened to, and validated in your fear. This advice should probably be handed out to Malady visitors at the border.

"When I say I feel lousy, that I'm going to die, just let me say it," Margie would instruct. "Don't give me this, 'Oh, no, you've got miles to go before you sleep' garbage. You don't know that.

"By the same token, when I feel great and make ten-year plans, don't bring me down with your own reality therapy. Sure, there's a fine line between all this, but it's mine to walk, not yours."

I told her she should write the manual. Although Margie seemed to have mellowed toward the variety of ways in which people deal with their major crises, she was still somewhat contemptuous of those who talked about "a small recurrence" instead of shouting "Metastasy!" as she did, the way she once boomed "Bob has cancer" or walked bare to the waist in the locker room.

In 1996, more than a year into her rematch with The Beast, she thought that metastatic disease was where first-time cancer had been in 1978, when so many people whispered that I had "The Big C" as if it were a death sentence and we ordered that reclining chair in preparation for my wasting away.

By the late nineties, people were living with metastatic disease for years, as they were beginning to live with AIDS. In the 1990 first edition of her breast cancer "bible," Dr. Susan Love did not write about metastatic disease. In her

1995 second edition, she apologized for the omission. She attributed it to her surgeon's bias of regarding metastasy as a defeat. As much as Margie liked the book, the sly skeptic in her wondered if Dr. Love had skipped the subject at first because metastatics didn't live long enough to buy books. Dr. Love had thought the possibility of recurrence was just too much to deal with while you are still struggling with the first diagnosis, too much of a downer to read about.

"I was surprised at the recurrence but not shocked," Margie would say. "I knew it was coming back. Tom Reynolds told me it always comes back. But I figured I'd be seventy-five."

In that first year after the diagnosis, there was a bone-marrow biopsy, outpatient surgery at the hospital that cost about $5,000 more than insurance covered. There would be wrangling over that bill for months. Worse was the result: There was cancer in the marrow.

There were "uptakes," or hot spots, on the coccyx and in the skull. But that was just bone, right, not spine or brain, she repeated to herself and us. Still, she slid down under the covers and sobbed, "I'll be dead by spring. Like Jackie."

When she slid out again, she considered the possibilities: alternative medicine, stick with Memorial, do nothing, travel, sue the internist she had liked so much—why had there never been scans before? Would earlier scans have found the disease at an earlier, more treatable stage?

"If she had been a fat, patriarchal, slap-on-the-ass male doctor, would I have been more demanding?" Margie would ask. "But she was so brilliant, a feminist, in the first woman's class at Yale."

The internist had tried to put a positive spin on the news. "Well, did you ever think you'd reach sixty?"

Margie was annoyed. Maybe back in 1981, at the age of forty-nine, newly diagnosed for the first time, she wondered if she would reach sixty. But once she *passed* sixty, she thought she was heading for eighty.

A woman who was diagnosed as metastatic from the start said to her, almost accusingly, "At least you had thirteen good years."

The gradations of it. Having cancer is like being a Native American or a Jew; the rest of the world may see you as part of a monolithic group, but if they don't know what stage, what tribe, what sect, how many nodes, they know nothing about you.

One of Margie's greatest intellectual strengths had been an ability to make associations, to lift out of a concrete situation and find historical, sociological, psychological, literary connections. She could weave a strand of local gossip with threads from Proust, Riesman's theories of individualism, and the latest songs and movies. Sometimes, it made for stimulating discussion and sometimes it seemed to distance us from a problem at hand. From the very beginning of the recurrence, however, at least with me, she was very focused on her own disease.

She moved back and forth between her "streetfighter" mode, in which she would growl, "No one's going to write me off," and a softer acceptance, in which she would say, wistfully, "I've had a good life, but it's sad not to see grandchildren. I'd like to live long enough to see Sam publish a book."

There were times when she didn't want a lot of sympathy. "I am a blowhard," she would say, instinctively understanding that the so-called "trash talk" of basketball players is not so much about psyching out their opponents as keeping up their own spirits. There were times she just wanted to cry. She could move between those modes in minutes.

Meanwhile, Margie's oncologist, Maria Theodoulou, kept offering good reasons for a positive attitude. She acted optimistic, warm toward Margie, tough on cancer, willing to keep trying different procedures and chemicals until she found the combination that would keep The Beast at bay.

ONE OF THE MOST positive moves Margie made in the months after her diagnosis was joining a New York City mutual help group for women with breast and ovarian cancer called SHARE. It had been founded primarily by middle-class, educated white women in Manhattan, many of them career professionals who transferred their portfolios from, say, corporate litigation to cancer. But by the time Margie joined, SHARE was reaching out to women of various economic, social, and ethnic backgrounds all over the city. The thrust was still toward support and education, but by lobbying for research funds, environmental laws, and health-care options, individual members were becoming politicized. It was very much the kind of feminist group that Margie had joined in the past, then fell out of as internal politics took precedence over issues.

She was steered toward a metastatic support group. She missed meetings because of radiation—members were always missing meetings for treatments and hospitalizations—but kept going back for the group's warm, no-nonsense attitude. Hearing about it reminded me of my old eighth-floor ball-team.

Through Margie I met and wrote about two SHARE members whose experiences qualified them as tour guides as well as fellow travelers in Malady. Odette Petersen was fifty-three years old, soft-voiced, nonjudgmental. Carol Hochberg was thirty-eight, quick and intense. They sat back to back in SHARE's spare Times Square offices several days a week, answering calls on the hotline. They listened to each other's phone conversations and passed notes.

Their own border crossings had been typical. During a regular mammogram Odette noticed that the technician wouldn't make eye contact with her. The radiologist said he suspected a small, early-stage, treatable malignancy. A half hour later, Odette was in her Manhattan apartment, a trembling hand on her telephone. She didn't want to call her husband, Rick, because he was in the midst of important business meetings. She remembered that nine months earlier, a friend had taken her to an Ann Taylor fashion show to raise money for a self-help cancer group whose name she did not remember. The group had a hotline. Through her chilly panic, Odette also remembered she had made a donation. Her hands scurried through her checkbook.

When the woman on the SHARE hotline answered, the first words that spilled out of Odette were, "I just found out I have a lump and I'm afraid to call up my husband and upset him."

The woman made a sound that seemed to signify she had heard this before, and could handle it. She asked: "Do you have a normal relationship with your husband?" When Odette said she did, the woman went on to tell her how common her reaction was, that among the many groups at SHARE were several for the newly diagnosed, as well as piles of books to read, lists of doctors and services, and, if she was interested, a place to be around women who could share the tears and the tumor humor. After fifteen minutes, Odette was calm enough to call Rick, who came home early, and then call a surgeon, who scheduled a biopsy.

Odette was on the hotline herself four years later when Carol Hochberg called and said, in a precise, hard-driving, power-lunch way, that she had a 2.5-centimeter Stage IIB tumor plus four positive nodes, and that she didn't want to call her mother and upset her. Odette calmly, gently wondered if Carol might like to be called back by a woman nearer her own age whose cancer was in a similar stage.

Carol was not typical of the estimated 184,000 American women diagnosed that year with breast cancer; she was younger (less than 10 percent are under 40), more affluent (a former investment banker), certainly more prepared to become an advocate for progressive changes in the medical and political approaches to the disease. She took a hard line, and held it, even after her cancer spread to her bones and liver.

"Little pink ribbons are not going to do it," said Carol. "Women have been conditioned to be ladylike, to be mediators, not to make too much noise. We have to get out there and kick; we can't take this lying down."

DESPITE THE DOCTORS' mantra—"Think spring!"—the winter of 1995–96 was hard on Margie, a painful, anxious, emotional roller coaster ride. Sam had moved in to take care of her. He was twenty-seven, a former rock musician settling into a full-time writing career supported by part-time teaching. He was single and his hours were flexible. Susannah, twenty-five, was absorbed by a job arranging for foreign high school students to live and study in the United States, and for Americans to go abroad. She often worked nights and weekends, but managed to spend a lot of time with Margie, often bringing along her boyfriend, Ben Nachumi, whom Margie loved.

Margie needed more and more help. At first, that meant getting her to and from outpatient visits. The definition of "help" soon expanded to include cooking, cleaning, shopping, and the management of drugs. Eventually, it embraced one of the most intimate and complex tasks a child can do for a parent—changing diapers.

But just getting to the hospital could be task enough. One Friday in February, Margie began screaming and flailing so much at the increasing pain in her back that Sam called her doctor's secretary, who arranged a private ambulette ($238 up front, we take plastic) to bring her to Memorial's Urgent Care. If you call 911, the ambulance will take you to your local hospital, which is probably not going to do much for your cancer treatment. As Sam and Margie later described it, two stocky women showed up at their apartment with a stretcher that could not be maneuvered into her bedroom. Screaming with pain, Margie stagger-ran out to the living room and fell on the stretcher. There was relief from the pain only while she was lying down, her weight off her cancer-riddled hips and legs. She was carried out to the elevator, but the stretcher was too long for the floor. It had to be tipped upright to fit. She cried all the way down twenty-two floors.

In the final scene of the agonizing farce, the two women could not lift Margie up into the ambulette. Sam had enough of his old high school shot-putter's muscles left to grab one end of the stretcher while they took the other end and hoisted it up. Then they drove her to the wrong hospital. Margie swore she was going to get her money back.

With Sam pacing nearby, Margie lay around Urgent Care most of that Friday, until she was admitted and shot full of morphine for the pain and Ativan for her anxiety. Margie could be a demanding patient, even querulous at times, and there is a tendency for medtechs to tune out such people for their own convenience.

We talked about it later as something Margie had to think through. At what point is it better for a patient to bite her tongue and lower the heat, just so potential helpers are not scared off? Dick Gregory had a parable about the value of comedy as a way of getting people to listen to his commentaries on American life. An old man falls down the stairs and breaks his leg. If he screams, people will run away and he will be alone; if he laughs, they will come to share the joke and stay to help him.

Margie had heard the story, in fact she had typed it from the transcript of my interview thirty-three years before, but she maintained that screaming vented her pain and made her feel better. If it drove people away, they probably wouldn't have been much help anyway, she said. I wasn't sure if she really believed that or was enjoying the debate. I argued that as long as you made potential helpers understand that you needed them, it was better to stay cool, to conserve your own energy and avoid flustering others.

At this point we were not all that sure what was causing her pain. Were the tumors on the spine getting bigger? Were there more of them? At worst, could a tumor be compressing the spinal cord, a situation that might have to be relieved by risky emergency surgery? Or, the most hopeful possibility, was she constipated from the morphine?

By that Saturday, she was mostly out of her head. Sam, Susannah, and I were there most of the day, and it was alternately horrible and hilarious, sometimes both at the same time. Given the right drugs, most everybody seems to hallucinate, but even there you get what you came with. Margie's hallucinations could be brilliant. Our favorite was her flight of fancy about the tattoos cancer patients wore on their backs: their charts, medical histories, drug dosages, doctors' notes, in blue and black and red. There was a starting point of reality, of course, in the blue dots that had been tattooed to target her radiation. From there she went on to answer out loud the questions she heard only inside her head.

Weekends are not the best time if you need information and test results in a major urban medical institution. The senior staff are in their country homes, and those with the duty tend to be young or inexperienced or angry at being there. The difference between constipation and spinal cord compression is considerable. The sweet young redheaded doctor, Sam's age, seemed to be betting on constipation, maybe because it was a condition she could handle. She forbade Margie to take food or water because there was danger of perforation. She described how intestines could literally explode, and feces spill into the abdominal cavity. There could be no enema for the same reason, she said, nor could laxatives be introduced by mouth, from the top of the body. The stool would have to be teased out slowly.

At least, that's what I thought she was saying. There is a tendency for young doctors to think out loud, to dump out memorized blocks of medical-school text along with their anxieties. Since it's our tendency to hang on doctors' every syllable and then filter it through our own faulty knowledge, the margins of misinterpretation are wide. You simply have to keep asking questions in Malady until you understand the answers.

An MRI was taken at 3:30 p.m., but no one was around to read it. All the radiologists were on their cocktail hour, I said to the redhaired intern. She quivered with a certain guilty delight at what she saw as the boldness of the remark, but then remembered that someday soon she would be one of them, not of us. But she had no clout; she couldn't pick up a phone and order the radiologists to work. At best she could only beg and cajole the residents into helping her.

Meanwhile, every six hours Margie was taking Decadron, a steroid, to treat the possible cord compression. At 8:30 p.m., no one had yet read the MRI, which would tell us if she indeed had cord compression and actually needed the drug. Also, the hospital wouldn't allow her to take any of her own pills, including the daily Prozac, for which she paid $2.50 per pill. The hospital was charging her $7.50 per pill.

Unable to bully out the MRI results, the redheaded intern finally flirted them out. There was no cord compression, very good news, but there were lots of bony tumors on Margie's spine. But what exactly did that mean, we wanted to know. Typical of weekends in Malady, the people who could answer the questions were not around. For example, no one had compared this latest MRI to the previous MRI. Were there more bony tumors than last time? Were they bigger? Why wasn't there a computer on every floor with access to every patient's records?

We caucused: Were these people lazy, or do they know something they are not telling us or are all the files in a mini-storage room in New Jersey and not immediately available? What about the basic questions: How much of her pain is from stool, how much from cancer, and how much does it matter?

In the midst of all this pain and anguish and doses of Dilaudid, Ativan, Haldol, Prozac, God knows what else, Susannah presented Margie with a bouquet of lovely yellow tulips, a beautiful and life-affirming gesture without question or edge. There is a reason for flowers in the hospital. Make Malady bloom!

And there are hospital moments beyond reason, impossible to understand, moments that must be hallucinations or part of a satirical movie, a medical version of, say, *Dr. Strangelove* or perhaps an episode of "The X-Files" in which people who work in these warehouses for the sick succumb to Mad-Nurse Disease.

In this particular episode, a very confident (bossy? insecure? insane?) nurse-clinician was standing at the side of Margie's bed reviewing the protocol before giving her a blood transfusion. The whole blood thing was fraught; the cancer was in her bone marrow, causing anemia, and one way that Margie took her own emotional weather report was by checking on her blood count. Above eight, she was feeling good, below seven, she needed more blood. The report was further complicated by how many units of blood she received, by how long she had to wait, and whether or not the blood was warmed for her, as Dr. Theodoulou ordered. The blood-warming machines were, depending on whom you spoke with, difficult to operate or old and cranky, and many nurses either did not know how to operate them or were too impatient.

Knowing that even the noise of a raised eyebrow could set off an overwrought medtech, Sam, Susannah, and I were flattened against walls to give this particular nurse-clinician all the room she needed to give Margie her blood. She began humming and grumbling and shaking her head as if she were arming a nuclear device to blow up the world.

We did appreciate her being careful and understood why she might be under greater pressure these days. New York State had recently issued a scathing report on Memorial's "systematic deficiencies" in communications and supervision after a neurosurgeon mixed up two patients and operated on the wrong side of one patient's brain. The neurosurgeon was fired, but it was hardly an isolated problem. After all, New York Hospital across the street had lost several patients, including Andy Warhol and Libby Zion, because it hadn't followed stringent-enough procedures. At Boston's famous Dana Farber Cancer Institute, a *Boston Globe* medical writer died after getting four times her prescribed chemo dose. There were always stories about wrong legs amputated, about surgeons going to lunch or to the airport to pick up their wives while leaving a patient opened up on the table. Sometimes Paddy Chayevsky's *The Hospital*, the opera buffa of tumor humor, seems like a documentary, where billing clerks hector comatose patients and doctors and nurses are so busy having sex they don't notice the patient dying in the next bed.

We were prepared to be very glad that this nurse was taking all precautions.

"No, it's not a match," she finally said. She showed us that the card that had come with the bag of blood read "Marjorier Lipsyte," rather than "Marjorie R. Lipsyte." While she admitted that the patient account number, date of birth, gender, race, and home address were all the same, it was more of a leap than she could take to assume that Margie's middle initial had slid over in some computer shuffle.

"You simply can't assume," she said, and the kids and I glanced at one another, remembering all the times we'd mimicked their otherwise wonderful third-grade teacher who always said, "Never assume, it makes an 'ass' of 'u' and 'me.' "

But what was funny at first because it was so dumb, became, because it was so dumb, horrifying. The nurse simply wouldn't allow Margie to get the blood even though it had been ordered and prepared and soon would spoil.

We argued, but carefully; she wasn't budging and we didn't want to make an enemy. What I wanted to say was, Hey, how is it that the smarties in billing are able to assume that "Marjorier Lipsyte" is "Marjorie R. Lipsyte" and keep charging thousands a month without worrying about that rogue "r" slipping out of place like the rogue cancer cells you are not stopping.

But we bit our lips and Margie cried and waited hours for a new card to be made up with the "r" now an "R." in the right place. The original blood had to be thrown away. Another bag was hung, but something was wrong with the tubes or the clips and it never dripped right and eventually it spoiled and two new pints had to be found, and it was almost twenty-four hours later that the transfusion was completed. By that time, Margie was a wreck and probably sicker than when the dark comedy began. We could tell that the medtechs were angry at all the extra work, but we couldn't tell if they were angry at the system or the downsizing or the Mad Nurse or at Margie for being the cause of all this trouble. We felt helpless. Not exactly sitcom material.

But a day later, we were all laughing, an ongoing lesson in even desperate hospital times. As with New England weather, all you can be sure of is change. Margie was sitting up, color in her cheeks, almost manic as she regaled us with tales of her "ten thousand-dollar shit." Using lactulose, she had cleared her system on a portable commode, which, of course, had not been totally cleaned, which was another story that was not exactly sitcom material.

A few days after that, back home, Margie began badgering the ambulette service by phone and mail until she got her $238 back.

I BROUGHT Margie a copy of *Time on Fire* by Evan Handler, a young actor whose battle with acute leukemia, first diagnosed in 1984, quickly became a harrowing and hilarious battle with the medical-industrial complex, most notably Memorial Sloan-Kettering. He went on to a much better experience at Johns Hopkins, where he received a bone marrow transplant for his usually lethal condition.

The book—there was also a one-man off-Broadway play—is a kind of guerrilla manifesto, bracing in its bold nastiness. But it is also so unrelenting in its attack on Memorial's "seething madness," on its uncaring clerks, nurses, doctors, even on other patients, that what might have been totally unnerving for a patient to read had it been more measured was a wonderful read just because it was so over-the-top. You could pick and choose what you wanted to believe and embrace. I loved his descriptions of the blood-work "vampires" and his shrewd ear for med-speak; when a patient gets sicker or dies, it is the patient "failing the protocol," not vice versa. His descriptions of chemo and cold-blood transfusions are masterly, and his sketches of his family and girlfriend under the awful pressure of his grave danger and of his constant neediness were easy to understand. The neediness itself, however, his thespian self-absorption, his lack of compassion for anyone but himself, were less easy to understand, although he forgives his universal cantankerousness—"I am a man impossible to please. It's what got me through."

The book had a distinctively feverish red-orange-yellow jacket that frequently caught the eye of passing doctors and nurses, who knew about the book and hated it. At first, Margie enjoyed their flinches, but after a while there seemed no reason to antagonize them, especially since Handler's awful experience was not hers. It was Susannah's idea to turn the book jacket inside out and print, on the blank white side, the name of that sweet children's classic, *Goodnight Moon*.

MEANWHILE, I KEPT waiting to get that call again from one of my parents. Dad was back at the deli counter within a few months, also driving around, climbing on the roof, raking leaves, shoveling snow. I wasn't exactly surprised at 7:30 a.m. on December 15, 1995, when my mother called, panic in her voice. Dad was in terrible pain in his chest and side. I said I was on my way, but to call an ambulance immediately. She wanted to wait for me, at least two hours, but I insisted that we meet at the ER.

In the cab to my car, I read in the *Times* about a sixty-two-year-old Manhattan editor and writer who had been indicted for manslaughter. He had helped his fifty-two-year-old wife commit suicide. She had been suffering from multiple sclerosis. The prosecution had used the honesty of his computer journals against him. He had expressed concern that his reaction to her intermittent calls for death was based as much on his need to be free of her as on her pain. He was feeling crushed under the burden of her care. I thought about that on the drive up, which led to a stream of consciousness.

First of all, I thought about the increasing burden on Sam. He hadn't complained, and I might also have been reacting to my own feelings of being something of an outsider in the care of Margie. Calls and visits are not the same as a day-in, day-out responsibility. Sam was living in Malady. I was a day-tripper.

Which led me to think that if this was it for Dad, what was I supposed to do? We had been lucky last time. My parents had taken care of each other for more than sixty-two years now, but Mom didn't drive and they lived in the country. There was no way I could do for either of them what Sam was doing for Margie. But could I do less? I was thirty years older than Sam. I'd probably end up with a heart attack. I thought of that because a friend had recently taken a stress-buster course after a mild heart attack and he described in great detail how your blood turns to sludge in a crisis. We were built that way, he had learned, so we wouldn't bleed out after being bitten by a saber-toothed tiger. I felt as though a paper cut could do that to me—even thinking about Sam and Margie and Mom and Dad. Why was I feeling so sorry for myself?

As I drove, I kept thinking about that assisted-suicide story. Theoretically, I do believe that people should have the right to select the time and the method for ending their lives. But the timing of the current debate made me uneasy. After years of hearing "Get a life!" we suddenly start hearing "Get a death!" Had this really come from people, or from economists and ethicists trying to wrestle health-care power away from doctors and hospital administrators?

Dr. Jack Kevorkian has probably done us all a favor by making us confront the issue, especially since more and more people are apparently committing suicide without him. The only death with dignity, some feel, is a planned death. Why undergo needless pain and expense?

The point at which pain makes life unbearable is a point that can be properly defined only by the person suffering that pain. Patients should be able to control their own morphine drips, and they should be able to turn themselves off forever.

And yet, the issue of expense keeps coming up. Who makes the decision that the expense is worthwhile or needless: a relative who is keeping you alive for an emotional reason or a relative who wants that money in the will? an administrator who wants to keep the profits rolling in from a vegetable or an administrator who feels there is more money to be made from a different patient using those facilities? a doctor hobbled by outmoded laws against pulling plugs or a doctor conditioned to believe that death is a doctor's defeat? a patient driven by pain or depression? a patient driven by guilt? a patient who doesn't know there is no hope? a caregiver who wants to offer a patient a death with dignity or a caregiver who wants a life of his own?

A physically vulnerable, emotionally needy person doesn't need a lot of clues to what a caregiver wants. A glance, a word, just the manner in which a pill is brusquely thrust or gently held out is enough to begin a train of thought that might end, Better for everyone if I were dead.

Margie and I had talked about suicide, tentatively, during our first bouts with cancer, and more comfortably, albeit still theoretically, in noncancer years when we routinely talked about everything in the news. The Hemlock Society, the deaths by self-asphyxiation of Bruno Bettelheim and Jerzy Kosinski, the emergence of Dr. Kevorkian, all kicked off discussions. Since we didn't keep handguns around, that was not an option. Despite the availability of fatal heights in New York there is something so violent and messy about jumping off a roof that it seems as much an attention-getting and guilt-provoking statement to survivors as an efficient way to end a life.

I had always wondered how many one-car "accidents" were suicides. Since taking a driving trip along the California coast, my own suicide fantasy had changed from swimming out to sea to flying off the rim of America. I would drive to the Devil's Slide in Big Sur, where the highway curves suddenly high above ocean waves breaking into spray against huge, jagged rocks. There was no guardrail above the Devil's Slide. I would stamp on the accelerator and steer into the clouds, then drop onto the rocks.

Margie had a scenario in which she would get into a warm bath, with barbiturates and bourbon, and cut her wrists. That became more complicated after we came to realize that to be sure of death a plastic dry-cleaner's bag pulled tight over your nose and mouth was necessary.

All this presupposed a physical and mental ability that no terminal patient can count on. The chances are good that one reason you might want to die is because pain and disability have made coherent thought and physical effort almost impossible. You can forget about taking yourself out when you can't even take yourself to the bathroom.

This is all from the patient's point of view. I hadn't started thinking about the survivor's point of view until I read *No Time to Say Goodbye,* by Carla Fine. I was casually leafing through it when the name Harry Reiss jumped off a page. I pictured the friendly, chubby urologist whose name I had written down in 1978 because I liked his bedside manner. I had actually been thinking about trying to track him down for this book. But he had killed himself in 1989 at forty-three.

"It was a very selfish act," said Carla Fine, his widow, when I went to see her. "People talk about the boldness, the audacity of suicide, but I see it as copping out. It's done out of fear and anxiety, not strength. The brave people are those who mop up the blood with Clorox, who clean the brains off the wall, who comfort the survivors."

Carla found Harry on his examining table, covered with blood. "Empty bottles of Thiopental were strewn on the floor, along with discarded needle packets, plastic tubing, and several Milky Way wrappers," Ms. Fine wrote in her book. "The IV pole was upright, tethered to Harry's waist by his black leather belt."

The police arrived and wrapped the office in yellow crime scene tape and interrogated her as a suspect, which is standard. She felt like a suspect for years, lying about the cause of death. Harry had a heart attack, she would say. It was in survivors' groups that Carla was able to express her anger, sorrow, guilt, and shame. Where else could she talk about the terrifying numbness, the financial problems, the stigma, the people who intimated she had driven her husband to his death? In a group, at the least, there was the comfort of a form of tumor humor. After one meeting, another widow who found herself being treated suspiciously by men, laughed and said to Carla, "Let's just go to a singles bar and set up three signs: 'He Poisoned Himself' and 'He Shot Himself' and 'You All Take Your Chances.' "

But why had he done it? Harry was the son of Austrian refugees who had settled in Cali, Colombia. He had his melancholy moods—Carla called them "black clouds"—but they passed and seemed a small enough price for a mostly happy life. The why of his suicide—both his parents, with whom he had a turbulent relationship, had recently died, but his urology practice was booming and his research papers were gaining attention—was, typically, an unresolved question overwhelmed by more painful questions. Didn't he trust me enough to confide in me? What else was he hiding? Wasn't my love for him enough to keep him alive? What did I do wrong? By the time she published her book, a survivors' companion, she had worked through her questions enough to realize there might just be no answers, no closure. When I met her, she was fifty, lively and funny, in a new romantic relationship. She spoke her mind directly about almost every current hot topic except physician-assisted suicide.

"That's a gray area for me," she said. "Are you ending your dying or your living? And what's the mental state of the doctor who is helping you? I can't forget that Harry's was a physician-assisted suicide."

As time went on, I sensed that Margie was becoming less interested in suicide as her condition became graver. This is common, and her streetfighter survival instincts were just too strong. As concerned as she was that the doctors would keep her alive as a vegetable, she was more concerned that they might kill her off, inadvertently or for their own convenience. Margie was always suspicious of power over her life in other people's hands. Who could be sure that an insurance company or managed care or even a Memorial bed counter would make a thumbs-up/thumbs-down, life-or-death decision based on anything other than cost effectiveness? In the raging debate over doctor-assisted suicide, what most people really fear is accountant-assisted suicide.

With all these thoughts going on in my head, the drive to the upstate community hospital seemed short. I arrived with my mind cooking. I was ready for almost anything except what I found. Mom was looking perky in a red beret and Dad was perched cockily on an examining table in a gown. They were smiling. It was just an attack of shingles, yet another virus Dad had never met before. Until the ER doctor had lifted Dad's shirt during the exam, no one had noticed the red splash of raised welts on his chest and side. Mom and Dad were feeling so good now that they were discussing at which diner they would treat me to a really large lunch.

THERE WAS MORE good news. Margie's markers were down. The consensus was that the Tamoxifen was working, that the cancer had not worn it out or broken through it. That may or may not have been true. When you don't have to make a decision based on an opinion, you might as well accept the optimistic opinion. Hope always helps. When Margie had a lot of pain in her bones, we liked to hear that she was having a "flare," a condition caused by Tamoxifen kicking hell out of the cancer.

"If I'm a good girl and take my morphine," Margie would say, "I'll have a life."

But thinking spring became an increasingly difficult act of will as the daily struggle with the advancing disease required more effort, took more time, emotion, and energy. Sam and Susannah would soon be overwhelmed. Margie would need private nursing and more home care help, which was a problem financially, logistically, emotionally. Home health-care workers are underpaid for what they do and typically undertrained, often exploited by the agencies that send them out. Many workers are recent immigrants on their way to better jobs. Some truly care, some are briskly professional, some are furious at having to do this work and don't care who knows it, including the patient. This is a growing problem for an aging population and needs to be addressed through more sensible insurance and Medicare coverage, especially as hospital stays are dramatically shortened. In the best circumstances, a patient makes a private arrangement with a strong and kindly nurse-nanny and they bond; this scenario, however, seems more like a TV movie than the reality, in which a different health aide shows up late each time. Punctuality is critical when ambulettes and procedures are waiting. Since Margie's insurance only paid for the aides to stay four hours at a time, for a limited number of days, scheduling their tasks was a task in itself. Sam and Margie could never be sure when an outpatient visit would end. One day I showed up at the hospital at noon to help Sam take Margie home, but her blood count was 5.5 and so another transfusion farce began. She returned home at 11:30 that night. They were getting used to it.

Two days later, Margie coughed blood and had chest

pains. After six hours in Urgent Care, she was readmitted to the hospital. Dr. Theodoulou was on vacation for much of that stay. A tall, gray-haired, middle-aged woman named Nessa Coyle, who was a registered nurse and a social worker, emerged as an important voice of reason and calm. She was the director of the Supportive Care Program in the Pain Service, which was in the Department of Neurology. When Margie heard—or misheard—casual comments by young doctors that sent her into a panic, it was Nessa, simultaneously commanding and compassionate, who could smooth the waters.

Once, an intern told Margie—or Margie heard—that she was being sent home for financial reasons, thrown out. This did not seem impossible. Margie had reached the limit on her insurance, and the drugs whipped her fear that her apartment would be sold out from under her to pay her bills. Sam called Nessa, who assured them it would not happen.

The offhand comments were killers, even when Susannah with her laser sharpness heard them. She was helping Margie through an endoscopy in day surgery when the doctors found erosions in her esophagus, caused by steroids, acidic food, eating lying down, and healing ulcers. When Susannah asked the young doctor about follow-up procedures based on the findings, he shrugged. "You or me, yes," he said, over his shoulder, moving away, "but she has too many other problems."

What other problems? With no time for discussion, how do we find out what he means? Did he mean first things first, we'll get to the esophagus later, or did he mean she was too far gone for treatment?

We could shoot from the hip, too: The reason you are so nauseated and dizzy, Margie, is because this new drug, Taxol, is really kicking butt; that's how you know when a drug is working, when it makes you feel worse. Who knows? Could be true. You have to keep spirits up to get through the rough patch to fight again. It's a cheerleader's job. Of course, you shouldn't be saccharine or off-the-wall with false chirpiness because that is the beginning of patronizing the patient, in a sense dehumanizing her, making her an object rather than the person you love who is fighting to live.

Dr. Theodoulou was good at offering hope. She had a new theory, based on a study somewhere, that Prozac can interfere with the chemo, actually act on the blood. Margie was to come off Prozac, which she had been taking for almost eight years. This raised all our spirits for a few days (and kept us busy speculating on how the loss of Prozac would affect her). Then a hematologist said that it was clearly the cancer attacking the blood. Meanwhile, Margie's left eyelid was drooping and for several days we thought she also had Bell's palsy. Then her eyelid snapped up. I was getting used to what Sam and Susannah and Margie already knew—there would always be something. As Reynolds Price asked, "What's next?"

IN A DELIRIUM, Margie called Nurse Kelly into her room with an urgent message: "Your husband said to say he was okay." We stood in the room bewildered, slightly embarrassed, as Nurse Kelly's face melted, as tears pooled in her eyes. She reached out for Margie's hands and thanked her profusely for "the gift." Nurse Kelly explained that her husband had been dead for seven years.

ONE DAY WHILE I was getting my monthly testosterone shot, a thirtysomething Fellow with an M.D. and a Ph.D. told me that the clinic had stopped dropping in those prosthetic testicles while the breast-implant lawsuits were in progress.

When my jaw dropped, he said, "Don't lose sleep over it, but be aware if the shape changes. Leakage could be an autoimmune disaster."

I tried to laugh. "So now I have to check a rubber ball for testicular cancer." When he started to back out of the room, I added, "That's tumor humor, son." But he was gone.

I told that to Margie. There were certain things she understood better than anyone else in my life. We laughed while knowing it just wasn't funny. I showed her a small item I had clipped out of a Herb Caen column in the *San Francisco Chronicle*. A business executive named Jim Easley, who had had both testicles removed, asked the doctor to place a zipper on the scar so he could keep spare cash and car keys in his scrotum. "The doctor was not amused," according to Caen, who was. Margie and I were too.

"SPRING" ARRIVED on April 10, 1996, Margie's sixty-fourth birthday. Susannah created a terrific party, which was briefly delayed because Memorial had its own birthday present for Margie, a port surgically installed under the skin high on her left chest for easier infusions of blood, chemo, painkillers. Margie was in Recovery when the partygoers—her brother, Bob, and his wife, Karen, Susannah and her boyfriend, Ben, and I—assembled in Memorial's lobby, which is a medical version of an airline gate area. Here staff members meet patients' family and friends to give them departure and arrival information. At about 6:45, an earnest volunteer told us with great assurance that Margie would be in Recovery past 7:30, which would then put her into the shift change period during which "nurses get very busy discussing their patients and sharing reports." We might as well go out to eat, she said; it would be several hours more before Margie would be returned to her room.

This was so at odds with what we had heard earlier that I glanced at the others with a quizzical expression. When the volunteer intercepted my glance, she said, very patronizingly, "I sense you are unsure of what I just said, so I will check again for you."

While she marched off feeling hurt, we all trooped upstairs to find Margie waiting for us in her room, very alert and happy. Another lesson: check it yourself; take nothing for granted.

It was a joyous party with cards, balloons, and birthday food. The handsome young knight-surgeon and his three merry young squire-residents came up to oooh and aaah over their port and to sample the different cakes. Being thin, moderate men, they were happy with small pieces, which they ate slowly.

After the doctors left, we immoderates had double helpings of cakes. Margie ate everything and then vomited neatly into a yellow plastic bucket. It was one chocolate splash. No big deal. I washed out the bucket without thinking about it. Later, when I did think a little about it, I was only surprised at how something that in another context might have been odd or unpleasant seemed natural, unnecessary for comment. Etiquette becomes Mediquette* in Malady. Such words as "manners" and "appropriate" and "offensive" and "distasteful" are best left at the border unless you are willing to give them new, loose definitions. There is no Emily Post-Op to make hard and fast decisions about what is and isn't "proper." Each traveling group must decide how it will deal with body parts and their juices and smells. You'll be surprised at what you can do when you have to. And sometimes proud of it.

I lingered after the others left. Margie had enjoyed the

* See page 239.

party. She said, "Glad you're here," which made me feel very good. My gift, a contribution toward the "think spring" laptop she was going to buy, led us into a reminiscence about the VTR we bought in 1978 in preparation for what we foresaw as my long and painful recuperation. Look how that turned out. But we were beyond bullshit and she was not optimistic. She did not think she would get to write too much on the laptop. Of course, she would be happy to edit what I wrote about her in my book. This book. She no longer had plans of writing her own book about metastasis. She reminded me that metastasis meant "other places," which she said would fit neatly into my own "another country" theme. She also wondered if I had made a note on her observation that the women in SHARE tended to call this hospital "Sloan," as if Memorial sounded too much like a cemetery. Or was it part of the hospital's public relations campaign? Sloan sounded jazzier, better suited for society columns. She suggested I check it out. Ever the editor. Seemed like old times. But there was such worry in her eyes.

"They just don't know what's eating my blood," she said. She wondered if this could be her last birthday. She might not make it to Medicare at sixty-five, she said. And she was very concerned about the mounting bills, which she thought could be more than $50,000 beyond her coverage. She sensed an increasing pressure from insurance and from the hospital, which was trying to get her on Medicaid so some bills would be paid.

Cancer improved our post-divorce relationship in the sense that it paved over so many of the bumps and potholes that otherwise would have made being together a jarring ride. We never talked about why we were no longer married; we made no attempt at all to resolve or even understand old conflicts. That was in a past that had no relevance to such a demanding present. We were totally focused on what athletes and their psychological handlers like to call "the now." You need to be "zoned" to win a game or to recover. So-called real life, even the solving of important problems, can be a distraction. This is why athletes, patients, and caregivers so often have re-entry difficulties after a prolonged journey in SportsWorld or Malady. Problems left to grow and fester may become too big to solve. Again, each traveler must decide how much baggage to take along.

Margie and I talked about cancer and we talked about the children in an easy, open, friendly, sometimes humorous way. I was the person on whom she knew she could most easily unload her concerns, the one person besides the kids she could be sure would come back for more.

They were handling the hard jobs—the logistical nightmares, the shopping, cooking, shlepping. Margie could be a very demanding patient, and Sam's response was to become a demanding caretaker: pills taken on schedule, an electronic alert system in case she fell while he was out, an attempt to organize daily life from bowel movements to TV-watching. There was a certain officiousness in his approach that I found remarkable in an artist, but also necessary for their survival. Sam was handling Margie well, even getting her to pipe down in the hospital; she had a tendency to speak too loudly about people who were in hearing distance (my parents shared that tendency) and to shout out for people. Sam's calmness calmed her, and his devotion touched people in the hospital, who would then reach out to them. There was a supervising nurse named Karen whose kindnesses—which included cutting through red tape—could bring tears to our eyes. The one person you really need, said Sam, is a nurse who gives you attention and comfort. That's worth writing on the sickroom wall.

Since Sam and Susannah were in charge, I decided my role would be to care for the caretakers, to support them in whatever way made sense, day by day, financially, morally, physically when needed. It's a secondary role that many people who can't be primary caregivers would be happy to take on if encouraged. Make sure the primary caregivers are eating well, taking breaks, tending to their own emotional and medical needs. Don't let them burn out, wreck their other relationships, lose jobs that are important to them. Caring for caregivers can be as simple as bringing coffee and doughnuts to construction workers or as complex as offering psychological counseling to disaster workers. My role was small. I mostly took the kids for meals and talked to Margie. She was often gloomy for good reasons—she couldn't have necessary dental work because of her condition, another home-care worker hadn't worked out because of attitude or a better job. There was a new drug, there was no improvement, the dunning letters and calls continued. Someone from the hospital had phoned to ask her what her apartment was worth. That upset her for two days. I said there was no way they would throw her out of her apartment, but then she wondered if after she died the hospital could make the kids sell it. I didn't know. I asked a lawyer, who said he could probably drag out proceedings for a while, but eventually they would have to sell to satisfy the hospital bill, even if Sam wanted to stay.

She was thinking spring but it was already spring and she didn't feel renewed. Every day she stabbed herself in the thigh to inject a drug that was helping the chemo work. The injections cost $650 a week; God knows how much the chemo cost.

I kept reminding myself that this wasn't even a medical horror story. We were getting the best care available, we thought, and we were staying alert. But when I stepped back, it was still a horror.

THE EMOTIONAL roller coaster picked up speed that summer, the dips and turns sharper every day. A bone scan showed more activity and the need for more tests, including a CT scan. The pain specialists moved in with one of the greatest advances in modern medicine—the simple philosophy that patients should not have to suffer. It was amazing how new this was. For centuries, perhaps because doctors rarely felt pain themselves, they were not concerned with patients' pain, downplayed pain so that patients were unprepared for it, and, hilariously, professed fear that heavy painkillers would make junkies of the old and the terminal.

Now, led by Nessa Coyle, the pain people told Margie to stay ahead of the pain curve by giving herself "rescues." These were little bursts of morphine she could fire into her IV by pressing a button, several times an hour. At home, she had extra morphine pills that acted in the same way. I wondered if this might be more psychological than actual, more of a placebo, some false sense of control over her pain. It was not as if she could give herself as much as she wanted, whenever she wanted it. And blissing out on morphine was no answer unless there were no more questions. You paid for that with constipation and a mushy head, and, eventually, with the end of all functions.

At the end of August we actually went to the hospital together, me for a monthly testosterone shot, Margie for a blood count to see if she needed a transfusion. I planned to hang out with her and take her home in the evening, but her count was high and when we left it was still morning of a beautiful day. We ate salads in a charming café and then walked and talked in Riverside Park, along the Hudson. The day exhausted her. Sam put her to bed and then he and I went out for dinner. A wonderful day, but it took her a week to recuperate, her stomach upset from the roughage of lunch, her bones aching from the walk. She told me that I had pushed her to do too much. I felt bad. Had I hurt her? It was a few weeks before I found out that I might indeed have let her walk too far, but that the problems were far more profound.

Through September, she was in much more pain, although her energy level was way up. She didn't need transfusions as frequently. But when she moved, her lower body screamed. Theodoulou was still in the game. "Maybe I can't cure you but I can treat you," she said, scheduling a visit to an orthopedist.

At the end of that month I saw an "NBC Dateline" show about that editor who had helped his wife die. It was skewed toward the opinion that he had killed her for his own convenience, not to end her suffering. The show depended too heavily on her relatives, who were very accusatory. They had had nothing much to do with taking care of her.

ON MONDAY, October 7, 1996, after what sounded like a torturous weekend hopping around on what turned out to be a fractured hip, Margie was admitted to the hospital for the last time. She had been virtually immobilized with pain after stumbling into the couch and falling against her side. The first priority was to control her pain. But she had become "toxic" on the morphine. The high level had tripped her into incoherence. And she was still in agony.

It was not clear how much Margie knew, or was able to understand. When I talked to her the next day, the dryness in her mouth was from the drug Dilaudid, which also made her sound dopey. She was giving herself a rescue every fifteen minutes. She was going through periods of confusion. She railed at Sam for not answering the phone at home before realizing that she had been dialing the wrong number for hours.

Nessa Coyle had told her that the morphine was no longer working, that it seemed to have run its course. During this hospitalization, they would try to find a new painkiller, perhaps methadone. There might be more radiation, especially since the tumors were advancing more quickly now.

There were more scans and more bad news. Her left hip was broken and her right one was eaten away. A surgeon wanted to do a hip-replacement operation, but Theodoulou said it was too risky in her condition. It also might be a waste of time and unnecessary pain if, because of the other hip, she would still be unable to put weight on her legs, to stand and to walk.

There was much discussion about the need for twenty-four-hour nursing care, about preparing for life in a wheelchair. Sam even learned how to ease her into a chair, using a board. He had wheeled her around before, but those were almost joyrides so she wouldn't have to walk or stand for long periods. She always got in and out of the chair herself. This was disability.

Theodoulou was still telling her to think spring, but since it was only the beginning of autumn, hope seemed very far away. Margie was depressed by the thought of the wheelchair, she told her friends Paul Gardner and Marlene Shyer, who were loyal callers. She was also thinking more about her internist and the bone scans she never had. We went back and forth on that. Sometimes she thought that earlier intervention might have slowed or even stopped the spreading cancer, and sometimes she thought it was better not to have known what was going on, especially if early action wouldn't have made that much of a difference. She might not have enjoyed that wonderful art tour, might not even have gone, if she'd known what was happening in her body. What we didn't know was whether or not early action would have made a big difference, and no doctor was willing to offer an opinion.

But Theodoulou did say that Margie should have been seeing an oncologist all along.

. . .

A PRIEST came in one day, a big, ruddy-faced Irishman with a *Going My Way* twinkle, and asked Margie what he could do for her. She thanked him but explained that she was not Catholic.

"No problem," he said.

She added that she was not particularly religious.

"Doesn't matter," he said. "So, how can I help you?"

She tried to wave him away, but he seemed so determined to do something that she finally told him, faintly embarrassed, that she needed someone to wash her face and then to shut off her light so she could sleep.

"That's easy," he said, and with a smile and a gentle touch, he washed her face with a cloth, dried it, kissed her forehead, shut off the light, and tiptoed out.

AS WE HAD for almost thirty years, we talked about the kids. Margie seemed resigned to not seeing them married and parents, but still sad about it. She told me that Sam was quite bossy with her, and when I nodded in agreement, she bridled at what she inferred as my criticism of Sam. No criticism of the kids was allowed, unless it came from her. I quickly added that Sam's bossiness was for her own good.

As it was, we had no areas of great disagreement, but I thought about how hard it would be if there were. It's a wonder how people handle the noncancer mucking and grinding of daily life when cancer looms over everything, dwarfing, trivializing, obscuring the life that goes on and still must be attended to.

All the drugs couldn't completely dull Margie's sharp mind. On October 8, she looked almost childishly innocent, her face round with prednisone and her legs swaddled in plastic sleeves filled with air to keep pressure on the blood vessels and prevent clots. We sat around, chatting smartly, like old times. All our spirits were lifted. That Sunday, Susannah and I went on a downtown Manhattan architectural tour. We had a good time.

When I called Margie the next day, we talked about Susannah, who had recently quit her job for several reasons, one of which was to take over Margie's care from Sam, who needed to get back to his writing and was in danger of burning out. Margie talked about how wonderful Susannah was, and how devoted, in terms she had used just a few weeks ago for Sam. Was she emotionally preparing for a changing of the guard? We played with that for a few minutes. Margie agreed that such a scenario was theoretically possible, but in this case she was just expressing her feelings. I wasn't so sure, and told her. She seemed to enjoy the give-and-take.

As it turned out, that was the last really long conversation we ever had. I hung up thinking she still had all her marbles; she was going to get through this patch, hibernate in winter while thinking spring.

I spent the next two days, Tuesday and Wednesday, following Muhammad Ali around New York in what was packaged as a community service tour but was really a publicity trip for a new book. Cycles again. I had started covering Ali in 1963, the year Margie and I got together. Other than my sister and my parents, Margie and Ali had been the most long-term, continual, important companions of my adult life. They met only once, in Sweden, where he was giving an exhibition in 1965 after winning the heavyweight title for the first of three times. In the fall of 1996, his star had risen again. Millions had seen him in Atlanta, shaking but confident, lighting the Olympic torch.

I had never, at least in my own mind, been either an apologist or a harsh critic of Ali, although I had been accused of both. But this trip brought out the skeptic. Here he was, suffering from some aspect of Parkinson's disease probably brought on by getting hit in the head so many times, trembling and fragile, led around by people who assured everyone that the champ was calling all the shots, even as they made all the speeches.

It was hard to give myself over to this trip to Publicity while my head was in Malady. What was happening to Margie seemed so monumental, so much tougher and grittier than anything I had ever been through or even covered, that to cover Ali, the biggest story of my career, without total honesty would be trivializing my own life. This didn't even make total sense when I first thought it. After all, what did one thing have to do with another? Why shouldn't one be totally honest all the time? But I did begin to feel a revulsion for the boys on the bus, from major TV executives to freelancers filing puffy stories, all sucking around Ali, romanticizing him, holding him aloft like a holy relic. Making money off him. As I was.

The bus trip triggered my own private seminar. Journalists are always trying, I thought, to break down the protective walls that their subjects put up so that we can have better, more intimate stories. Meanwhile, we build our own walls between our lives and the stories we cover. Some of that is professional, to make sure that self-interest and emotions don't color our reporting, but much of it is personal. Less so in sports, which is mostly about staged entertainment, but certainly in the coverage of everyday people in crisis, the reporter is in danger of being sucked into a pool of unsolvable problems. Like a doctor with a failing patient. We have our defenses, our escape hatches, our skepticism, our smart-aleck comments.

There is only one person in my life who can truly understand all this self-indulgent philosophy, I thought, who knows me and the stories well enough, and she is half-mad with pain and drugs. I was already feeling her loss.

MY COMEUPPANCE for running around like a sweaty young reporter after Ali, with a dose of righteousness yet, was to come down with a lousy cold. I didn't know if it was the actual running around or the change in weather or having not gone to yoga class in several months. Short on cash, I was going through a cheap phase. But I used the sick-time in bed to read a wonderful new book, one of the very best about a real human response to disease, *Seeing the Crab: A Memoir of Dying*, by a therapist in San Francisco, Christina Middlebrook. She wrote about angers and fears, about sisters who called and those who didn't, and how enraged she became when she told people that she had metastatic breast cancer and had undergone a bone-marrow transplant and they, in response, started talking about their arthritis.

But what endeared her to me was her take on the New Age health hustlers who imply that serious disease comes to those who deserve it, who bring it on themselves by some issue or attitude festering beneath the surface of their lives.

"Thus," wrote Middlebrook, "because I got cancer in my breast, I must have been too maternal, or maybe not maternal enough. God save us all!!"

She came to understand "the gimmick," which was that "healing," to Bernie Siegel et al., "does not refer to a cure, which is what I wanted, but to an attitude to accompany me so that I can smile my way through this vile disease. I think dying is difficult enough without having to achieve a pleasant attitude in the process."

I knew that paragraph alone would be worth the price of admission to Margie, but I wasn't sure about the entire book, with its uncompromising view of metastatic cancer as an eventual killer. Margie herself had articulated that view when she'd been feeling good at home, but I wasn't sure it was a book she would want to read at Memorial. There would be time enough when she was discharged from this latest skirmish. I read the book carefully without marking it up.

In any case, I wouldn't be bringing it over so soon. I knew better than to walk onto a cancer floor hacking and sneezing. I called her on Saturday, October 19, 1996, to tell her I wouldn't be visiting that weekend. Shamed by mere sniffles, I upgraded my cold to the flu.

"I have something much worse," she snapped. "A pain in my sternum."

We talked about the pain, which she thought was caused by tumors. She said it was more painful emotionally than physically. Her blood was up, she had needed no transfusions lately, and she felt energetic enough to be imagining herself scooting around in the chair, wheeling around the apartment on her own, cruising Broadway and Riverside Park with some help before winter set in, and, of course, thinking spring.

This new pain reminded her how fragile were her plans and her good feelings. I started a pep talk, but a doctor came in and she had to get off the phone.

I I

THE LAST WEEK of Margie's life was a kind of gift to the three of us, an intense time, spiritually, emotionally, and physically. For six days and nights we gathered, often with a half-dozen friends and relatives, at her bed as if we were sitting around a campfire. We told stories and jokes, listened to music, ate meals, slept. It was a very intimate time, and it brought us all very close. Margie was the campfire, and we warmed ourselves at the flickering flame that was her life.

HER DYING began sometime in the morning of Tuesday, October 22. Sam called, his voice urgent: "Mom's had a massive heart attack. Better come quick."

While I deny being a supernaturalist, I've already admitted being a sucker for signs and portents. It was spooky for me to recall the decision I had made the day before, a Monday, to write and to file my column for the Sunday City section. I never file that column before noon on Wednesday, for two reasons I consider important: One, always give yourself until the last minute for late-breaking events and, two, don't let the editors get used to early copy should you someday need that extra time.

But on Monday, after a weekend in bed trying to keep a bad cold from becoming the flu, something told me to finish a column I had already begun on my junior high school re-union, not to wait until I felt better. When it was done, a voice told me to file it immediately. Electronic transmission takes all of two minutes—what's the rush? But the voice in-sisted that I clear the decks, have one less thing to worry about. I sent it in, not sure why it seemed so important to get it out of the house. By the time I reached Memorial that Tuesday afternoon, I knew why.

Margie was slipping in and out of lucidity, sometimes in the same sentence. A tube coming out of the wall behind her head carried 100 percent pure oxygen to her nose and mouth. She was talking through the plastic mask. The heart attack seemed to have surprised the doctors. She was gasping for breath when Sam called in a nurse, who called the doc-tors. An EKG confirmed a damaging attack. "Ischemia" was the word they used. Not enough blood was getting to her heart, which in turn was not sending enough oxygen to the lungs, which were working too hard. Margie, a lifelong swimmer, had a powerful heart and lungs; even at diminished capacity they were probably stronger than most.

The doctors didn't know that then. The cardiologist was prepared to move her to intensive care, but Theodoulou made the decision for "comfort care." This was in keeping with Margie's wishes not to be resuscitated and to avoid dying in pain.

We talked that afternoon. Drifting in and out of lucidity, Margie the great talker, the recreational conversationalist, smart and quick-witted, put on her last display of that in-credible memory not only for detail but also for the connec-tions between people and events. When she called Sam "a Martian," as weird and hallucinatory as it seemed, I was sure there was a logical core; somewhere they must have read in a book or heard while surfing the tube or just riffed in a late-night talkathon that "Martians were the jailers of the ancient world." Sam's recent more authoritarian form of care made him a jailer, thus a Martian.

My favorite Martian. He held her hand and stroked her cheek and kissed her brow, weeping, crooning, "Don't be scared, Mom, don't be scared."

Even now she could be funny, bending words and thoughts. She talked about being "free-mated" after her death and recounted a dream—a hallucination?—about a Mrs. Lipsyte and school and an event called "fan-night surprise." My mother's first name was Fanny. There was something almost mischievous about Margie in this state.

The hospital kept sending up hospital food, gray hamburger wheels and swampy brown soups, but custard was all that interested her. We were beyond commenting on the food. There is something almost willful about the crimes of hospital nutrition, the hidden calories and sodium, the refusal to attempt to match meal to patient, and the way that food deliverers bang the trays down, daring them to be eaten. In the hospitals of the future, there will either be real nutrition or kitchenettes so family and friends can prepare food that has some connection to health. For the moment, however, the energy spent railing at hospital food is probably better spent just replacing it with take-in.

We were beyond nutrition. Sam and Susannah sent me out for Margie's favorite ice creams—Häagen Dazs French Vanilla and Ben & Jerry's Strawberry Kiwi sorbet, which she did not like separately, but mixed in proportions that only she and the kids knew. I scoured the Upper East Side neighborhood around Memorial and finally decided they were probably West Side flavors. I didn't want to risk being out searching for ice cream while she took a turn or died. I came back with the closest flavors—Häagen Dazs Vanilla and Ben & Jerry's Cherry Garcia. As it turned out, it didn't much matter. She was beyond taste, sad for someone who had so enjoyed eating.

She tried to speak. "I just want to say . . . wait a minute," but no logical sentence would follow. I wondered if she had had a stroke, if blood wasn't getting to her brain.

By Wednesday, a hard core of regulars had formed: Sam and Susannah, myself, Ben, who sat quietly in a corner carving a tiny soapstone statue for Margie, and three close friends of Sam's, Marion and Mike, who were engaged to be married, and Cynthia. They often arrived together, carrying food and gifts. Marion brought Margie a Curious George doll. For days it perched on a pillow above Margie's head watching Marion rub lotion into Margie's feet, a wonderfully useful comfort and one of the loveliest of gifts.

I began referring to the three of them as "the house band." Sam did not like that, and snapped something about trying to see them as individuals. At first, I attributed the crack to his ragged nerves, but eventually figured out that it wasn't all his problem. They were a family to him (Sam's memorable line was "Family is who shows up"), and I must have felt outside that circle. The three had often been at Margie's apartment, ate and watched TV with her, and Marion had also become a frequent phone pal. Marion was a force, an attractive, bustling, thirty-six-year-old blonde with a stage presence—she was a comic actor. It took me a while to feel comfortable with them—Marion mostly, since Mike and Cynthia, as warm and lively as they could be, still hung back until called up. As much as anyone, Marion was keeping the room alive, feeding the campfire with stories, movement, sheer energy. She had experience at this; her mother had died at Memorial nine years before, of brain cancer. Marion had taken care of her in her final months. She made no secret of the connection; she was both reliving that event and giving it a new, improved draft. And once I got over my own petty sense of jealousy and displacement, I learned from her. I began to tell stories around the campfire.

In 1970, before Susannah was born, when Sam was two, the three of us went to Newport, Rhode Island, and stayed in a large apartment the *Times* had rented for those of us covering the America's Cup yacht races. Margie had carefully marked "SAM" on a container of milk she put in the refrigerator, but the milk in that container and in the next few containers kept disappearing faster than Sam was drinking it. It was a mystery until she caught one *Times* reporter filching it for his cereal and coffee. She caught him in the act of pouring, and she screamed at him, "How can you steal a baby's milk?" He pretended not to get it: "What's the big deal, why you making a federal case?," but she did, and he finally shrugged and walked away. We didn't see much of him for the rest of race week. He made an effort to come in late and leave early. We laughed at that. Margie the she-bear. Steal her baby's milk?

You remember that, Margie?

We held her as we talked, our fingers inside her curled hands.

That was the summer Sam began to talk, and among his first words, while strolling the Newport waterfront, was "Want boat, want boat." He kept pointing at the yachts in the harbor. So we took a sightseeing cruise. After fifteen minutes, as the boat reached open water, Sam suddenly bellowed, "No more boat," and bolted for the rail.

You remember that, Margie?

She might tighten the grip.

"Thanks for the squeeze, Mom," Sam or Susannah would say.

Margie's brother, Bob, showed up. Of his three older sisters, Margie was the closest. I liked Bob. He was smart and lively. He taught math in high school, blew the trombone, and loved watching football, which he had played well. Margie had once expected him to win a Nobel Prize, or at least revolutionize the math curriculum. In this time of her dying I think he recalled her disappointment. As he left that day, he said he didn't think he would be back, it was all too upsetting for him. But he kept coming back with his wife, Karen, and stayed for longer and longer visits. He called often. Despite his own pain, he reached out to Sam and Susannah. Family is who shows up.

I usually dressed up when I was going to make a hospital visit. On weekdays I would wear a tie and jacket, on weekends, something a little more casual, but still what my generation calls a sports jacket. I began that habit in the late sixties and early seventies, when Margie spent about ten days each in the hospital for her three cesareans, and then in the early eighties for the mastectomy. Dressy but cheerful clothes, a way of decorating the room. Margie always liked that.

There was another reason, of course. Having started at the *Times* as a teenager in the late fifties, I tend to still dress in Journalism Conservative—blazers, dark suits, tweeds, like a lawyer who isn't going to court that day. I don't think it's a bad idea to give doctors and nurses the impression that even if you aren't a lawyer, you probably went to college with a few. It's not about threatening malpractice or even accountability, it's about class; the M in M.D., besides standing for Medical and Money, also stands for Middle Class. Like it or not, it's a fact of life that doctors speak differently to people they consider on their socioeconomic and educational level. The older doctors tend to be patronizing enough to everyone; who needs to give them more reason to treat you like a case instead of a person?

In extreme times like this, it is the nurses, not the doctors, who make the difference. Nurse Jane, a favorite of Margie's, moved her into a private room. It was the right thing to do, but we weren't sure that was the entire reason. A rumor had panicked us. An intern had said that if she stayed this way for any length of time, she would be moved to a hospice, but all we heard was the word "hospice" and we imagined the move was imminent. For a few hours we were upset that she would be disturbed. Her noisy, labored breathing could not be pleasant to any roommate on the other side of a thin curtain, and all her guests (Sam and/or Susannah slept over every night, on the floor or in a chair) were an imposition. We never found out if it was hospital policy to move her or one humane nurse's choice or whether it was done because someone expected her to die soon anyway. Nurses stopped taking her vital signs.

Three of Susannah's high school friends from New Jersey, Laura, Cathy, and Kim, showed up. It was tough for them. They all had mothers Margie's age, and they all remembered Margie as a larger-than-life presence in the household. But they quickly caught the spirit of the room, and helped pump up the volume, talking about their studies and careers, as if Margie, in what seemed to be a drug-induced coma, could understand. One of them remembered being thrown out of the house one evening ten years before. "You have to go home now, Cathy," shouted Margie, "I'm punishing Susannah." They all laughed. Margie squeezed a finger. Thanks, Mom.

Typically, it was also a time for the misunderstandings brought on by ragged nerves. People have to be very careful what they say in such charged times, and everything has to be heard through a kind of filter, taken with many grains of salt. While it seemed as though we should all be on the same page, all focused on Margie struggling for breath in that bed, we were each also constructing our own reactions to the scene. My mother, unable to get into the city, felt out of the loop. She called Kathy, who was working very hard at making it easy for me to be with a family that did not include her, and said: "No matter what you do, it will be wrong."

My mother understood immediately how terrible that sounded. She tried to smudge the hard lines by explaining that she was trying to say that Kathy was in a difficult position and that she shouldn't worry about anything. But even-tempered Kathy—always ready to force a dutiful smile—was upset. After all, she had become deeply involved in Margie's dying by supporting my involvement. Kathy gave me the time and the psychic space to be somewhere that had no place for her. Sometimes helping means stepping aside, getting out of the way and putting your own needs on hold.

One of the best things Susannah did was to decorate the room with photographs, to make it Margie's room. One picture, Margie looking gloriously windblown on cliffs near Big Sur, fit neatly over the small screen of the hospital TV that swung out over the bed. Tuned to a channel that broadcast a classical music radio station—there was a bluish TV light but no picture—the photo was back-lit and Margie glowed. I found it necessary to subtly—perhaps not so subtly—remind everyone that I had been on that trip too. Who do you think took the pictures? I didn't want to be out of the loop.

There is a very strong case to be made for family care, for a patient hearing familiar voices and being touched by familiar, loving hands. Why shouldn't you bathe your spouse or mother or sister? Why should it be a low-paying, devalued job for a poor woman who can't get anything else? Blood and brown discharge leaked from Margie's mouth and nose. The doctors were not concerned by it, so the nurses cleaned it off and suctioned her mouth only when they were asked. We could do the job, and we did. It was easy and made us feel good. We had no other patients to attend so we could make a loving, crooning ritual out of it.

My sister, Gale, arrived from California. A Jungian therapist, it took her a little time to become part of the campfire. A calm, low-profile personality, she was more used to directing groups than being in one. We talked about how much more we could learn to do. "Why is it that only so-called primitive people in undeveloped countries take care of their own?" Gale asked. We decided that once managed care figures out how much can be saved by free family labor we might have more humane medicine.

A thirty-one-year-old intern, Dr. Francis S. Lee, joined a small group of nurses in our pantheon. A thoughtful, gentle man who had a Ph.D. as well as an M.D., Dr. Lee was not only kindly in his approach but also able to explain matters medical in clear terms. He explained that Margie was in "multi-system failure." She was profoundly tired. Her heart was not getting enough blood and was working desperately hard, as were her lungs. Her body was shutting down to concentrate energy for the heart. Meanwhile, as the regulated parts of her system were responding to the energy-saving shutdown, the unregulated cancer cells were running wild, growing, interfering with circulation and organs.

How much longer did she have?

"Modern medicine can't answer that question," said Dr. Lee. He would say that more than once those final days.

There was a bent sense of time in that room crowded with loving caregivers, littered with books and sandwiches and pictures and Indian food and soda bottles and plastic containers of hardening ziti. Time passed so slowly, so intensely. It was the richest of times. We spoke to one another over those gasping, groaning breaths, but always kept one ear open, like a radar shell, for any change. Late one night, all of us dozing around her, I fantasized the boatmen on the river Styx trying to drag Margie into the boat for the voyage out. She was not ready to go, and they couldn't budge her.

We talked as if she could hear, and I suspect she could. Once, a relative standing by the bed began asking about Margie's condition—"So, is there no hope?"—and Sam directed him to either speak to her or speak outside the room. When I said something about funeral services, Susannah told me not to speak negatively in the room, that we were trying to keep out all jarring or scary thoughts. Susannah was right. Nothing scary. Sam kept crooning, "Don't be scared, Mom, we're all here."

I told Margie I was still trying to get the book she wanted, Claire Bloom's *Leaving the Doll House,* about her years with Philip Roth. I reminded her of our one Philip Roth story. Many years ago, a good friend, then about twenty-one, met him at a literary party and went home with him. She never told us the details of that night, but she admitted they were potentiated by the fantasy of literary parties on the arm of a star. But when morning came, Portnoy/Roth opened his eyes and said, "On your way out, could you dump the garbage?" Then he turned over and went back to sleep. I couldn't remember if she had actually taken out the garbage. Margie would have remembered.

The caregivers took care of one another. Sam's friend Rob brought apples and chocolate, a great energy-boosting combination. Marion, Cynthia, and Mike kept handing out vitamins. Because we had no idea how much time Margie had, no one wanted to take a night off, to leave for a real meal or a hot bath. It was enough of a break to go to the lounge to laugh at a sitcom or walk around the block talking about something else.

Outside, in the city, other dramas were unfolding. The Yankees were going for their first World Series championship in eighteen years and the manager's brother was waiting in another New York hospital for a new heart. Even to a sportswriter, the baseball story seemed fabricated, synthetic. Real drama was in this room. Real drama was the skinny young man who went downstairs to York Avenue for a smoke, the drip bags of chemo hanging from his rolling IV caddy. He stood on the sidewalk, a hospital gown over jeans and a teeshirt, smoking and puking and talking to a young woman who could be his girlfriend. He was wearing a Yankees cap.

A reddened bump appeared on the right side of Margie's head. Susannah felt it while stroking her, recoiled, wept, and called for our wonderful Dr. Lee, who explained that it was "consistent with a contusion." Perhaps there was a fracture in her skull from one of the tumors, and blood was rushing to the site. There was a pained hopelessness in his eyes as he reassured us, "I don't think it is hurting her."

What a difference a Dr. Lee makes. But he was only the mop-up doctor, the relief pitcher who comes in after the game is long won or lost. The real cancer doctor, the warlord in the battle, as Sam called the optimistic, up-tempo Maria Theodoulou, was absent. She had fought the good fight and kept Margie's spirits up and cried "Think spring" to get her through yet another rough patch. Now she had retreated to crank up her energies for those she could save.

(A few weeks later, I mentioned this to a former Memorial doctor who knew Theodoulou well. "The good ones have to do that," he said. "They have to distance themselves from a patient's death, or each time they will die a little too, and soon there will be nothing left of them.")

But as Theodoulou retreated, the nurses moved in. The difference in function between doctors and nurses is never more apparent than at such times. Doctors treat the disease. Nurses treat the patient, and the family if necessary.

Nessa Coyle came in and touched Margie with her long, elegant fingers. "Rest your body and your soul," she said.

IT WAS MY JOB to arrange for the cremation; I was grateful for the task. Making calls, gathering information, was enough like what I ordinarily do to offer a kind of normalcy. After three days of what we had finally come to accept as a death watch, I could go out.

The first calls I made were to the brand-name funeral homes where I had gone, with increasing regularity over the years, to other people's memorial services, one on the East Side of Manhattan, one on the West Side. I had no idea at the time that both had recently been bought by the world's largest owner of funeral homes, a Texas company with a large share of the high-end New York market. The people I spoke with at those two funeral homes, on the phone and in person, were subdued and professional. There was no false sympathy. I appreciated their directness, which made it easier to question the prices.

A basic cremation cost between $2,700 and $3,000. The funeral home would pick up the body from the hospital, then hold it under refrigeration until a family member came to make a visual identification and go through an estimated 1½ hours of paperwork. Then, accompanied by a "licensed funeral director," the body would be transported out-of-state in a "limousine" to a crematorium where bodies were cremated "individually." This turned out to be a key word; the upper-end funeral homes implied that when several bodies are processed at the same time, you can never be sure exactly what is coming back.

The "cremains" would be available about four days later. An urn for the ashes would cost anywhere from several hundred to several thousand dollars; a casket for a memorial service (which cost about $1,200) could go as high as $29,900. Solid copper.

There was something comforting, mesmerizing, in these calls; somehow they distanced me from the impending death, from dealing with grief. The numbers and the language were numbing. It was suggested at the high-end places that I create an "expects" file with them, but I said I would call back.

I called two places picked out of the Yellow Pages. At the first, a man with an Anglo name and an office in Spanish Harlem spoke with the insinuating smoothness of a good car salesman. He said the total cost was $410. All his company did was cremations. Three business days to return the cremains; for an extra $125 I could have one-day service. He dismissed my question about group cremations, of getting other people's remains mixed in with mine. There were state laws about procedure, he said, which everyone followed.

"Then how can you explain," I asked, mentioning one of the top-end funeral homes, "the disparity in price?"

"I get this question all the time," he said. "You are going to have to ask them why they are so expensive. There is no rationalization."

The other low-end place, in SoHo, was $399. They offered a room for a memorial service for $200.

The day after I gathered all this information I stumbled into a funeral home near the hospital, a somber but not unpleasant place. There were pamphlets on grief, free calendars and pens. An enormous, friendly young man who overflowed his desk handed me a sheet of paper with a price list, and went over it. Cremation was $995. I liked him immediately, but wondered if I was just cutting the difference between the high and low ends. We chatted. He said he was the fourth generation in the business that bore his great-grandfather's— and his—name, John Krtil. He said his immigrant great-grandfather had been a blacksmith in Eastern Europe who had probably made coffins, too. That became his trade in nineteenth-century New York. He said this was "the only independent funeral home on the Upper East Side."

He explained that cremation would be in a combustible cardboard box that left little residue. Remains would be returned in another cardboard box. He advised against buying an urn if there was any possibility we might want to scatter the ashes.

I asked him about the more expensive funeral homes. "They are thieves," he said.

And the cheaper ones?

"Even in the very best of circumstances, there can be residue. If the circumstances are not of the best . . ." Krtil shrugged.

No visual ID would be necessary, he said. If I filled in some of the blanks now, the paperwork could be cut down to a few minutes when the next-of-kin came in to sign permission for cremation, a state law. He said to call when we needed him.

SLOWLY, WE BEGAN to realize that Margie, a person who always wanted to get to the party early and leave it late, was being kept alive by the energy in the room, by the stories and the laughter and the crooning, "It's okay, Mom, we're all here, we love you," and the touching and squeezing, and the music, mostly classical on WQXR, the *Times* radio station that she loved, and loved to mock. ("They're not allowed to play Mozart in the morning because the publisher once cut himself shaving to *Figaro*.")

A nurse had told us that people sometimes "slip away" when loved ones leave the room for a while. While none of us would take responsibility for letting Margie go, it became important in our minds to give her the chance to let go if she wanted to, not to hang on for us. We were all pretty ragged by now, especially Sam and Susannah, who had had little sleep. Susannah's face was a clenched red fist and Sam's face was puffy and blotchy, presumably from something picked up while sleeping on the hospital floor.

We decided that everyone would try to get a good night's sleep on Sunday night. Bob Rubin's last words to her were "I'm leaving now, Margie, I'm going home to watch football and play Dixieland." That was his loving little joke. If anything would wake her up, shouting with big-sisterly advice, it would be that. She couldn't stand his passion for football, and she thought he spent too much time on the trombone.

Before I left I was briefly alone with Margie, and I told her to go rest if she was ready, that everyone had said what they needed to say, or as much as they could say, that we all felt satisfied for now. I told her how Marian, a nurse she liked a lot and had called "first-class," said it was "unbelievable that she had fought so long." Margie would have liked to hear that. I told her how our beloved Dr. Lee was gone—rotated off the floor to something called "night float"—and how Marian was going to have to break in another intern who would be gone by the time he or she learned the procedures. I told her how Marian and Dr. Lee and others had said they had been touched by the dedication of her visitors, how they felt the love in the room.

And then I surprised myself. I told her I still loved her, and that I would see her on the other side. Our conversations were not over.

I HAD SLEPT for an hour when Susannah called at 12:30 a.m. Margie had stopped breathing. A nurse had taken her pulse and announced that she would be gone in another few minutes.

After Susannah made the call, Margie took a huge, gulping swimmer's breath. By the time Gale and I got to the hospital, her breathing had resumed, a labored, ragged snore, but strong enough now to keep her going for hours more, said the nurse.

We arranged ourselves around the bed. As the oldest, I got the recliner this time, and tried to doze. At 4:30, Gale and I went back home. Fiftysomethings can't pull all-nighters.

MARGIE DIED somewhere between 7:40, when the nurse last took her pulse and went for a doctor, and 8:00, when the doctor declared her officially dead. Sam was the only one of us there. Soon after Gale and I had left, it was decided that everyone would leave. Sam, especially, needed a hot shower and to sleep in a bed. He was downstairs on the street, smoking, saying goodnight, when he suddenly decided to go back upstairs. He had slept in her room every night since the heart attack; why should he leave now so close to the end?

He climbed into the recliner, slipped on a Walkman headset, and holding Margie's hand began to drift off. The activity at the bed around eight o'clock woke him up. When the doctor turned to him and shook his head, Sam wrapped his arms around Margie's legs and began to sob.

He called us. "She's gone," he said. Gale and I rushed back uptown. After so many glorious Indian summer days of bright sunlight streaming through her hospital window and cool, starry nights, the weather had turned bleak, with chilly gray rain pissing down.

Sam said that the most awful sound was the final whooosh as the nurse turned off the wall unit sending oxygen into Margie's mask.

By nine o'clock she was yellow and waxy.

There was a tentative knock on the door. An elderly worker asked if he might come in. He just walked to the head of her bed, and looked down into her face. As we watched, a single tear began to roll down his dark, creased face. He touched her arm through the sheet, then looked up at us. "We used to talk when I cleaned the room," he said. "She talked to me."

When he left, I went to the rain-streaked window and began to cry.

SAM WROTE the paid obit that appeared in the *Times* two days after Margie died.

> LIPSYTE—Marjorie. 1932–1996. Editor, journalist, activist, novelist (*Hot Type*). Died on October 28, after a battle with breast cancer. She was the loved and loving mother of Sam and Susannah, beloved sister of Bob Rubin and cherished friend of her former husband, Robert Lipsyte. A woman of fierce love and lavish feeling, of compassion, wit and hope, she gave to us in her life, in her dying and in her death, everything.

Susannah and I made only one change in Sam's draft. He had used the adjective "heroic" before the noun "battle," and we thought the word was a cliché, especially since it's used for every ballplayer who comes back from arthroscopic knee surgery. He agreed, and we thought of "courageous" and rejected it. We tried to find an adjective that would include her qualities of being stalwart and uncompromising before we decided that we didn't need an adjective there at all; it would only diminish the word "battle."

It was a lively, warm, English-majorish discussion, just the kind that Margie had reveled in for many years through so many books, columns, reviews, school reports. I kept thinking she would pop up with a word and a very definite opinion on why it was the only one to use.

I WAS EXHAUSTED after we came back from signing the cremation papers at the John Krtil Funeral Home and reserving the room for the memorial. I hadn't realized how much energy is thrown out at such a time, even if most of what I did for a week was sitting and looking at a person in a bed.

Now, with nothing specific to do, my strength ran out. The cold and sore throat that had been dogging me for two weeks, that had kept me from visiting Margie the weekend before her heart attack, flared. I had just enough energy the next few days to make a few phone calls. Mostly I watched TV and slept and read about death and dying. I had bought Sherwin B. Nuland's *How We Die* and Harold Brodkey's *This Wild Darkness* weeks before, but had only looked them over.

Nuland, a doctor, wrote an amazingly clear description of just how the body begins to shut down as organs are starved of oxygen. We all shared copies of his book, and understood the process that Margie's heart attack had accelerated. "We rarely go gentle into that good night," he wrote. "Death is the surcease that comes when that exhausting battle has been lost."

Brodkey, a brilliant writer of fiction, wrote about his own dying in a series of edgy observations. He even tried tumor humor when his doctor offered to arrange tranquilizers and therapy to soften the shock and despair.

"Look, it's only death," responded Brodkey. "It's not like losing your hair or all your money. I don't have to live with this."

He admitted that he wanted to make them laugh, to make them admire him. He also didn't want to be pitiable, or to suck all the air from their world. He had once been impressed by a man who had fought hard to get well, until the man's wife confided that his long battle was killing her. The struggle dominated their lives and, wrote Brodkey, "he was hardly alive except as a will to struggle."

THE MEMORIAL SERVICE was held at the Riverside Chapel on the Upper West Side of Manhattan, because it was a few blocks from Margie's apartment, where a reception would be held afterward. I arrived first, almost an hour early, nervous that the event would not be a success, that few people would show up. We had picked a room with hard pews that seated about eighty, which seemed optimistic, an airy room with sprays of green flowers painted on white walls. It evoked Margie's "think spring" mantra.

I was relieved when the kids appeared; they clearly had a grip. For background music as the guests arrived, Sam had selected Mendelssohn's Octet in E-Flat Major, a favorite of Margie's, which he said, in his eulogy, "makes me think of spring, too, with its quick beauty and sunniness layered over a deep sadness, a sadness of knowing winter will come again." Susannah had ordered a magnificent display of yellow and purple flowers for the front of the chapel.

I was very proud of the kids. I was not surprised that Sam could pick music or write a moving eulogy or that Susannah could pick flowers or the food for the reception. But I didn't know until they did it that they could organize and supervise, in the midst of their sorrow, a party that their mother would have loved. The room was packed, a perfect fit of mourners from every stage of her life, from an estranged older sister through old *Times* friends, feminist colleagues, later SHARE friends, and, from the final months, pals of Sam and Susannah who "chilled" with her and sometimes crashed in the apartment. Half a dozen spoke. I did not. What could I say? I had left this woman. I was married to someone else. Margie's last two years, her final battle, revealed her essence. How could I praise that honestly without either sounding like a reporter or explaining why we were divorced? I wasn't going to spill out in front of this crowd. And, honestly, I still don't have the answers.

My eulogy wasn't missed. And one paragraph from Sam's eulogy captured everything I could ever have hoped to say.

He began by describing the emotional topography of the hospital room.

There was a great energy and love in that room, and it was emanating from her, and flowing through us, and gave us the strength to overcome our own fears, our own weaknesses, and stay, and be with her. I remember at one point my Uncle Bob turned to me and said, "She is teaching me so much," and I was thinking that same thing the whole time, too. She shocked doctors and nurses with her toughness, her refusal to yield, to give ground to Death. She did not shock those of us who knew and loved her. In the true sense of the phrase, Death took her. She did not go.

12

EVERY FOUR WEEKS I return to Memorial for a testosterone shot. Other arrangements could probably be made, a nurse-practitioner nearer home, the new daily skin patch. But I feel a certain umbilical relationship with the great gray stone building, a comfort in the connection. Although I don't see a doctor every month, I do see a nurse. I could always ask her about a troubling symptom. I do not consider myself cancer-free. My bad guys are in the woods setting up ambushes. So far, my good guys have been keeping them at bay.

Since Margie's death, Memorial seems less forbidding. It showed us a human face. Nessa Coyle, the pain lady, called a few days later to see how the family was doing. So did our favorite intern, the beloved Dr. Lee.

Two months after Margie died, I had lunch with my own doctor, the bouncy Paul Russo. He had been a Fellow under Willet F. Whitmore and I was fascinated by this link between my two surgeons, two handsome, energetic men with the gift of sweeping their patients along in their aura of confidence.

I met Russo at noon, at his office at the hospital, a small space crammed with books, monographs, computers, and decorated with photographs of his wife and small daughters. His nurse/assistant, Susan Alfano, my usual shot-giver, was in one corner, using a chair as a desk. In another corner, his chair touching Russo's, a medical student was setting up a database, twenty years' worth of kidney cancer patients cross-referenced by treatments and outcomes. I was surprised at how cramped and makeshift the conditions were for such important work, and surprised that such research didn't already exist, instantly accessible for every urological disease. When I mentioned this to Russo, he just rolled his eyes. Even this was possible, he said, only because of a grant from the foundation of a grateful patient.

He took me downstairs to meet his wife, Mary Sue Brady, a general surgeon specializing in melanoma. Her office was decorated with photographs of him and their small daughters. A pretty woman, Brady was as reserved as Russo was extroverted, although she was excited by a recent triumph. An HMO had refused to pay for a procedure Brady had perfected, which she insisted would save a forty-year-old melanoma patient. Despite the insistence of its own doctors, the HMO maintained that the procedure was experimental, and therefore not covered. But Brady and the patient had kept up the pressure—letters, phone calls, appeals to medical and government groups—until the union through which the patient was insured took an active interest. The person in charge of benefits threatened the HMO that the union would transfer its 5,000 members to another health plan unless it paid for the procedure, which it did. Brady had just performed the surgery, and the prognosis was good. It was the kind of victory that Brady wanted the world to know about. Even in these critical times, if you keep fighting you can win.

Russo was uncharacteristically quiet as his wife spoke. He beamed, he shifted from foot to foot, but he was quiet. I was almost as fascinated by this glimpse behind his white coat as I was by Brady's story. More than fascinated, really. I was . . . thrilled.

Almost forty years of interviewing people—famous people, reluctant people, a few dangerous people, sometimes even on live television—had given me a protective, professional cool. But there was something about being inside this life-and-death world that recalled the excitement of the days and nights with Bullets and Cloudy. No wonder cop shows and doctor shows are such TV staples. The intensity of the lives of these characters, the high stakes, our dependency on them, turn their fires into infernos. And add to that, I was watching my very own surgeon.

Russo took me downstairs to get his coat from the Operating Room Surgeons' locker room. It could have been in a YMCA, rows of red metal lockers, wooden benches bolted to the concrete floor. Surgeons wandered past in their green gowns, hair caps, cloth masks dangling from their necks. They checked their beepers, gossiped, made calls from a single wall phone. They sat at Formica tables in a small, shabby room with food vending machines, drinking coffee and eating sandwiches. It was noon and some of them looked exhausted. Pros after a tough scrimmage.

"Pretty fancy, huh?" said Russo.

"I've seen better locker rooms for community college football teams," I said. What I wanted to say was, So tell me about each of these all-stars and what are they doing and can we go watch them work?

On the way out of the hospital, we kept passing patients of Russo, and he had a word and a shoulder pat for each of them. "You get that aneurysm checked, Horace; it'll kill you before your prostate does." Russo had been at Memorial for more than twelve years, and he was doing about 500 operations a year now. He was a major producer; each of those operations generated how many tests, procedures, office visits, hospital nights, work for other doctors, nurses, medtechs? In Malady's new economics, he might be more important to Memorial than the Nobel Prize–winners it used to try to recruit. And his personality might be as important to his success as his skill. It was easy to like and trust him, and confidence in your doctor is the mojo of healing.

He was relaxed and expansive at lunch in a pleasant, upscale Italian restaurant nearby that his wife had recommended. He told me that his father was a urologist in Ithaca, New York. ("He's C. Paul Russo—get it, See Paul Russo," he laughed.) They sometimes talked shop on the phone. Once, after performing an orchiectomy, the elder Dr. Russo had sent the patient downstate to his son for further treatment. It was a proud moment for both of them.

The younger Dr. Russo had considered pediatric oncology until he came under Whitmore's influence. Whitmore proved you could be dashing and competent, accessible and a pioneer, said Russo. Unlike many doctors of his day at Memorial— and, apparently, of this day as well—Whitmore was beloved by his Fellows and assistants. He made sure that younger men were appointed to important committees, were sent to prestigious conferences, were groomed for leadership. Russo said he wanted to be like Whitmore. Well, not entirely.

One summer evening several years ago, Russo told me, he was sitting in a park near Memorial holding his eight-month-old daughter, Grace, cooing to her, bouncing her in his arms, when Whitmore spotted them through the fence, walked in, and sat down. Whitmore had just come from the annual party of the hospital's twenty-five-year club, and had had a few drinks. Grace reached out and touched his face.

"Who could resist that face, so handsome and kindly," said Russo, his own boyish face softening. "And I'll never forget what he said to me. 'You're doing the right thing, Paul. I didn't spend enough time with my kids. I'm trying to make it up with my grandkids.' But, of course, there wouldn't be much time. He already knew he was dying of prostate cancer."

. . .

THERE MAY BE only one person in my life who can truly understand my feelings about illness, Memorial, my doctor, one person who knows me and the back stories as well as I do, and she is dead. I think about Margie often. Several times I have almost reached for the telephone to share something with her, read her a paragraph from the book. I know Sam and Susannah go through this every day.

Margie never wrote her own book, although she bought the birthday laptop. Susannah remembers the day they shopped for it as one of the last really active, nonmedical days they had together. She cherishes the memory of that day and urges people to get out and share pleasures while they can. But she also remembers happy, funny moments when Margie was in bed, at home or in the hospital. On every level, from complete recovery to death, the trip to Malady is what you make it.

While Margie lay dying, Sam said to me, "I never thought I'd be doing this for one of my parents before you did it for one of yours."

"You've taught me how to do it," I said.

CANCER IS A TOUGH act to follow, even if it only roughs you up a little. It's a conversation-stopper among noncancer folk, and even within the tribe it gets complicated. Through a neighborhood group fighting a noisy bar, I met a man with multiple myeloma who said his doctors gave him four more years to live. From my questions he had figured I had battled The Beast myself. When he asked me what kind of cancer I'd had, I felt like the Army Reservist who never went past basic training and summer camps talking to a Vietnam vet. I started babbling something about having had just a wimpy little cancer. He, in turn, told me not to be ashamed of my cancer; he knew people who had *died* from testicular. At that point, we both recognized how surreal the conversation had become, and we backed off and returned to discussing ways to operate on the noisy bar.

The power of that word. The old paperback *Roget's Thesaurus* on my desk has three synonyms for cancer—hydra, curse, plague—and then refers the reader to the entry "wickedness." But given the choice, I would much rather have had my two cancers than Roger's diabetes, the Crohn's disease that has dogged Godie since childhood, or the progressive neuromuscular disorder called Charcot-Marie-Tooth disease which has been progressively atrophying the muscles below the knees of my friend Susan B. Adams. Susie, a gifted writer and editor, was a rising young tennis player when this rare form of muscular dystrophy was first diagnosed. Now in her forties, she walks with a limp and hits "the wall" of fatigue without the graduated warning signals most of us receive. Her disease is not life-threatening and it is not particularly visible. Navigating in this "shadowy world between illness and health" has its own special problems.

"Sometimes I even think it would be easier to be clearly disabled," she has written. "At least then there'd be no pretending, no denial, no need to put on a cheerful face."

Putting on a cheerful face takes an enormous amount of energy, and even for a pretty, prideful jock like Susie it is mostly about making other people comfortable. It is only recently, through a support group, that she is beginning to give herself a break, to stop trying so hard to appear "normal."

Like so many people living heroically with multiple sclerosis, strokes, or heart conditions, Susie winced sympathetically when I first used the word "cancer." I'm not sure I've ever convinced her that she is walking a tougher road than I am, and that I have much to learn from her stubborn courage. Malady is a big country and we are often strangers to our fellow citizens.

A friend in northern California, who had gone through her own painful and anguished medical ordeal in an unsuccessful attempt to become pregnant, asked me recently if I had a "cancer knot" in my stomach. It was a good question, and to give myself more time to answer it I pretended not to fully understand.

Cancer knot?

A constant fear, she explained, a looming dread.

Finally, looking out of the vaulted windows of her fine house into the woods, I answered the best I could.

"Not at this moment," I said.

THE WORK IN progress continues. Margie's ashes are in a closet of her apartment. We are still waiting for the final accounting of her bills. Susannah is in a grief-therapy group; she says it is very helpful.

An old friend calls to break a dinner date. His wife doesn't feel up to it, after all. The lump on her breast, aspirated a few days earlier, has just been biopsied, and the good news has been rescinded. It looks more serious than the doctors first thought, but they won't know for sure until they see the pathologist's report. So, no dinner tonight. My friends just want to hide and hold each other.

I miss the stop signal and plunge ahead. Are they reading Susan Love's book? Will they go for a second opinion? Are they satisfied with the flow of information so far?

"So far we're getting too much information," my friend says. "They give us the first drafts and the second drafts and the ad-libs and their own thinking out loud."

We will keep in touch.

Of course, I'm not necessarily the one they might want to keep in touch with, since my stories don't all have happy endings. But I call back a few days later. The pathologist has confirmed the bad news. We are soon exchanging tumor humor.

They are in the thick of the fray now. She tells me that her mood has changed for the better even as she still awaits results of bone scans and CT scans and the audience with a famous oncologist.

"That first week I was cleaning up the house for my husband's next wife," she said. "This week I bought myself a color printer since I'll be doing more work at home."

Margie would have liked that.

MEDIQUETTE

A Traveler's Guide to the Country of Illness

THIS IS NOT the last word. I keep adding to it, from my own experiences and from the experiences of friends, family members, and interview subjects with cancer and too many other diseases, and I'm sure you can add to it as well. In fact, please send me your notes, tips, and comments. I can use all the help I can get.

My traveling days aren't over.

I. DEALING WITH THE NATIVES

1. Doctors

Even as a new generation of doctors with sensitivity training and lowered income expectations stumbles out of medical school prepared to feel our pain, managed care has managed to make it more difficult for them to hear us out. The doctors often have quotas to meet, and shorter office visits are one way to help meet them. Although so-called gag orders are illegal in many states, HMO doctors are often restricted in what they can tell patients about procedures and protocols that may not be covered. Just when the battle for accessible medical records is being won, patients have had to fight harder for vital information. We have to be smarter and tougher.

Remember that the doctor standing before you is a professional technician trying to be compassionate while not being burned out by the needs of hundreds of sick people, some of whom won't get well. You can assume that doctors will minimize your potential pain and suffering, with the rationale that increasing your anxiety will only hamper your progress. And doctors will tell you what they think you need to know—and what they think you want to hear.

So—decide what you need and want to know. Prepare to get it and then to deal with the information. You've heard all this before, but it can't hurt to hear it again.

Go to the doctor with a written statement of your medical history and your immediate complaints. Go with a list of questions, a notebook (even a tape recorder), and a friend or family member who will also listen hard and take notes. You don't have to be aggressive; in fact, you should be tactful and pleasant. You are dealing with another human being, a partner in your healing. But be firm and focused. Don't leave until your questions are answered and you understand those answers. Better, smarter doctors will appreciate this approach because it means fewer problems, including lawsuits, and less time to spend in the future correcting misinterpretations of misunderstood information.

Knowing what you need to know includes the information to make a decision about treatment that fits your life. If the suggested chemo may leave you deaf, and you are a musician, push the doctor to find a drug that will only ruin your golf game.

Remember, doctors really do want you to get well. They just don't want to go broke in the process.

2. Nurses

A nurse I know who edited the house organ at a major California hospital set up a feature in which a nurse and a doctor would switch jobs for a day and write about it. The nurse had a great time—it was like a day off, she said, with a decent lunch hour and coffee breaks. The doctor was exhausted. He'd had no idea how hard nurses worked. And how different their functions were. He thought they were just there to pick up after him, like Mommy. He was unaware of nurses' own very substantial body of philosophy, history, and technique.

Simplistically, for starters, remember that doctors are supposed to cure the disease while nurses are supposed to treat the patients, which often includes their families. There are many specialists among nurses, and nurses have aides and helpers for some of the housekeeping duties. This all breaks down pretty quickly in a busy hospital. Nurses tend to be overworked and underpaid, certainly compared to doctors, and under constant pressure.

This means we have to cut them some emotional slack and handle them with finesse while demanding service. ("Should this hurt me so much?" is one way of calling for a long-awaited pain pill.)

But it also means we have to check their work whenever possible. Make sure that is *your* name and the correct dosage on those medicine containers and IV bags. This is not always so easy to do while you are sick. Often it's a job for your visitors, your caregivers.

All this checking applies as well to the various blood-workers, lab personnel, technicians. Try to be smooth about it if you can, but mistakes can be fatal.

And here's a tough one: Make sure all who touch you wash their hands first. Staph infections in hospitals are very common and busy people don't always pull on fresh gloves between patients. This is not easy to notice or to demand, but it is worth the effort to at least be aware of the danger.

As Sam said, the one person you really need is a nurse who gives you attention and comfort. When you find such a person, hang on for dear life.

3. Gatekeepers

The border guards of Malady, those receptionists, clerks, and secretaries, can be bridges or barriers to medical service. Be nice, be firm. Practice what was called "sly civility" by the colonials trying to get what they needed from their British rulers; excessive politeness as you march steadfastly forward. Ask for what you need—that appointment, that call-back, that test result—in a pleasant manner. But make it clear you will keep coming until you get what you want.

You are a patient, not a prisoner. You are not being punished. You have an absolute right to be at least as angry in an unresponsive medical setting as you would be if your car was being mistreated by a mechanic. You are paying for all this, one way or another. And it is their job to serve you.

HOSPITALS HAVE patient advocates. Some are public relations reps, some are real ombudsmen. Call them if you need them. Call the medical associations to complain, the state agencies. One good aspect of the current "mangled care" disorder is the increasing interest in customer service. Medical people are disturbed at the way patients are "shopping around." They call it disloyalty. I call it consumerism. Make it work for you.

And when things do work for you, let people know about it. No big gifts or tips—these are professionals, after all—but a thank-you note, flowers, candy, a book to doctor, nurse, or other helpful person is never out of line. People like to know they are appreciated. They deserve it.

II. PACKING YOUR HEAD FOR THE JOURNEY

The baggage you've been carrying your whole life is the baggage you will carry into Malady. The trip may ultimately change you in some important ways, but the way you initially approach your illness—with bluster or submissiveness, denial, confrontation, optimism—will set a tone to which others will react. Try to be aware of the image you are offering, not necessarily to change it, but to understand why you are being treated in certain ways. Are you seen as a passive, accepting LOL (medical jargon for a little old lady) or as a "krock," complaining about everything? Be who you are, but if you are an LOL or a krock, you may sometimes need someone else to intervene for you with medical personnel.

You certainly have a right to be angry at being sick, but it's a waste of time and energy unless you can use that anger to get information, to exercise, to make yourself better. Go with whatever works for you. Some people plunge into their work or hobbies to avoid "giving in" to their illness, others "get into" their illness as a way of understanding and fighting it. It's your call. Just remember that sometimes the stress and frustration of trying to act "normal," to pass for well, may make you sicker or at least hinder the healing process.

And here is a personal prejudice: Don't swallow too many self-help books on an empty mind. I find nothing as sickening as perky pep talk like, "Cancer starts with Can, not Can't," unless it is the pseudo-religious arrogance of the "Will Yourself Well" bedpan evangelists. The evidence is mounting that the causes of illness are generally found in biology, not pop psychology.

And it never hurts to let your attitude give you a lift. 'Tude saves, I say. Tumor humor is medicine too.

III. RATES OF EXCHANGE

Money was once a dirty word in Malady, at least in the mouths of patients, but since doctors and hospitals have begun aggressive advertising campaigns, we can at least feel free to ask about fees in advance.

Shopping by price for a doctor is not always wise—it's the flip side of hospitals making cost-efficient rather than medical decisions—but it's not a bad idea to let your "health-care provider" know you are concerned about money. Adjustments can be made, especially if you are paying all or a large portion of the bill. Savvy medical consumers negotiate these days. If you are willing to pay the entire bill up front and then go after the insurance reimbursement by yourself, sparing the doctor's office the chore of filing a claim and waiting for it, you may be able to get a discount from that doctor.

Getting reimbursed, even more than getting well, is basically the patient's responsibility. And so is making sure that your bill is accurate. At the very least, read it over as carefully as you would a restaurant bill. Of course, it's easier to challenge the shrimp cocktail you didn't have than the blood transfusion you didn't have, but then the shrimp was so much cheaper.

Keep a dated log of all your office visits, tests, and procedures in a basic bookkeeping pad or in your computer. Record amounts charged, paid, when insurance claims were sent out, reimbursements, follow-up calls made.

In the hospital, if you can, keep a list of the doctors who see you, who merely stick their heads into the room, the medicines you are given, even the paper products you are given (you may be charged extra for that Kleenex). This is difficult, especially if you are doped or sick, so get help from visitors.

Always insist on an itemized bill. Check and question it, promptly. There are often deadlines for challenging bills. Don't be rushed into payment if you aren't sure, and don't hesitate to call the hospital, the doctor's office, the HMO, the insurance company. Be nice. Be firm. Be back tomorrow.

There are private companies that will audit your health bills for a fee. A trade organization, the National Association of Claims Assistance Professionals, Suite 102, 5329 South Main Street, Downers Grove, Ill. 60515, can make referrals if you can't find any in your Yellow Pages under Insurance or Medical Claim Processing Services.

As usual, it's best to interview before you hire. You want someone with experience either in claims work for an insurance agency or as an insurance processor for a doctor or a hospital. It's like wanting a tax lawyer who once worked for the IRS.

I know you've heard this before (in this book, among other places), and probably ignored it before (I have, still do), but here goes: *Read your insurance contract.*

And while we are talking money, let me intrude just a little further into your private life. If you also happen to have twentysomething kids who are too cheap, too poor, or too carefree to insure themselves, do it for them if you can. You know you won't sit by saying "I told you so" while they get second-rate service. An appendectomy, no complications included, can easily run $15,000. A simple sarcoma can cost you the house.

IV. LEARNING THE LANGUAGE

You will probably never be totally fluent in medspeak unless you go to nursing or medical school. But you can probably learn enough to read your own chart and eavesdrop in hospital corridors. At the least, when medtechs are talking about "crispy critters" or "gorks," you'll know they are referring to burn victims and patients in vegetative comas. A GOMER is usually a messy nuisance (it means Get Out of My Emergency Room). You are a "pt.," and "stat" means right away. There are many glossaries and dictionaries available in libraries and bookstores. Among those worth checking out are the *American Medical Association Encyclopedia of Medicine,* the *Merck Manual, Physicians' Desk Reference,* and *Merriam-Webster's Medical Desk Dictionary.* This book's excellent copy-editor reports that the *Encyclopedia and Dictionary of Medicine, Nursing and Allied Health,* published by W. B. Saunders Co., is excellent too.

In the past several years I have subscribed to more than a dozen of the estimated thirty health newsletters published by medical centers from Baltimore to Berkeley. I find they tend to cover the same topics within a month or so of one another. I keep reading about restless leg syndrome, the possible powers of garlic, and the options in treatment for prostate cancer. So just pick one or two general ones, then find ones in your particular area of interest.

The National Health Information Center, P.O. Box 1133, Washington, D.C. 20013-1133, has a list of toll-free phone numbers for health information.

For Web browsers, the Internet seems promising as a source for research and for fellow patients, particularly for rare diseases and those with complicated treatment options. The February 1997 issue of *Consumer Reports* has an excellent article about Web sites, "Finding Medical Help Online."

The National Library of Medicine (http://www.nim.nih. gov) maintains MEDLINE, a computerized database of articles that have appeared in 3,800 biomedical journals since 1966.

Even if you can't understand your medical records, always get them (you'll find someone who can interpret for you). The records belong to you. The Public Citizen Health

Research Group, 2000 P St., N.W., Washington, D.C. 20036, can help you get your records.

The most patient-friendly book I've read, and one I highly recommend, is *Take This Book to the Hospital with You,* by Charles B. Inlander and Ed Weiner. It's smart and breezy, and it has a travel guide format that makes it an excellent Malady companion.

Sharing information with other patients is risky and rewarding. In a hospital waiting room or an Internet chat room, you can get a life-saving tip and you can catch a misinformation virus. Support groups with educated facilitators are safer. Then again, it was in a casual conversation that author Reynolds Price, after several years of suffering from swollen legs, found out about the Jobst extremity pump.

IV. TOUR GUIDES AND TRAVELING COMPANIONS

Malady can be dangerous for the lone traveler. But you can't count on safety in numbers either unless the people supporting your journey are working together, and in your interest. You can be sure that a serious illness will rearrange some of your relationships. Fast friends will unfasten and pull away; others will surprise you with smart, concerned care. Let people help you. Assign them tasks if you can, duties during a doctor's visit, flower arranging, shopping, walking your dog, a foot massage, medical research. Everyone can do something, most would like to, and many need guidance because they are simply unsure and afraid. Appoint a spouse, close friend, or colleague, who can act as major domo and coordinate your "volunteer tour staff."

While you are the patient, the center of attention, the star of the show, you are not going to have a long run if you burn out your caregivers. Yes, you need most of your energy for your healing process. But you don't stop being a person just because you are a patient—express your appreciation, don't make unnecessary demands (don't be a power patient!), and make sure those people taking care of you also take care of themselves and one another.

Caregivers should call or write Well Spouse Foundation, 610 Lexington Avenue, Suite 814, New York, N.Y. 10022-6005; (212) 644-1241, (800) 838-0879, for support and information. Its slogan, "When one is sick . . . two need help," is a valuable diagnosis.

If you are in the hospital and day-tripping visitors simply need to do something, let them tidy up the room. But be sure it is you or your designated aide who decides whether someone charges out to the nurses' station to scream for a long-awaited painkiller or just goes to buy cookies so the night nurse will drop into the room more often.

V. A PERMANENT HOME IN MALADY

1. The Personal

Chronic diseases that require long-term medical care may also require some long-term readjustments. Your relationships with your body, your environment, your family and friends may undergo enormous changes. Anxiety, fear, and depression are common, often indirect results of the disease itself, *direct results* of the rearrangements. A social worker, therapist, or support group can help you understand what is happening and how to deal with it. Proper nutrition and regular exercise are more important than ever. Yoga is the best combination I know of range-of-motion exercise and relaxation technique. You don't need a swami. There are books and tapes on so-called bedtop yoga.

Experts think that worrying about pain can sometimes be as debilitating as the pain itself. Modern pain services prescribe drugs to relieve that anxiety. The best course of action, and one that is becoming more common as pain control is becoming more sophisticated, is enough painkiller given early enough. The latest trend is toward "preemptive analgesia," in which painkillers are administered *before* surgery, which lessens post-op pain.

Pain is real; it is not in your head. You don't need to suffer. Your chances of becoming hooked, even on morphine or methadone, are slim since you are taking them for specific physical, not psychological, reasons. There are no free-lunch painkillers—they have their side effects too. You should be prepared in advance for the duration and intensity of them.

For all the debate about physician-assisted suicide, whether it promises death with dignity or is the slippery slope toward managed murder, most patients seem to cling tenaciously to life as it ebbs away. Survival is in our genes. In any case, for the sake of your family and friends, make your wishes known in advance and write them down.

Call it compassion, I call it cutting slack. Malady is a hard place. Sometimes people act badly, or at least not as well as you would like. The process of grieving, for a lost limb, lost vitality, a lost loved one, cannot be quantified in managed-care minutes. Ordering a person to "Get on with it" or "Snap out of it" is probably as helpful as a slap in the face. Give people the space and the time to work out their senses of loss. It always takes more time than you think.

2. *The Political*

No one wants to become a professional patient, but there are larger issues that have impact on our care. Do we continue to compete with one another for the shrinking medical face-to-face time or do we band together? As "cases" and "units" and "diagnostic codes" we are easy to ignore and manage. And we are often so fragmented by disease interest groups that we can't help one another as fellow customers and citizens of Malady. As well-meaning and helpful as each foundation and society and institute may be to its constituency in the short term, one wonders if each individual battle for attention and research funds doesn't hinder the broader course of effective, accessible health care for all.

Imagine the irresistible force of all the groups dedicated to AIDS and arthritis, to the different cancers and birth defects, to heart disease and spinal injuries, not to mention the rare afflictions that often get lost in the shuffle of money, joining forces for all who are sick. You can bet that the politicians, the doctors, the hospitals, the drug companies, the HMOs would listen and respond to a Patients Union. Maybe it's time for a bedpan revolution, or at least an organization really dedicated to the needs of the sick and to those who love and take care of them.

Count me in.

THE MAJOR FLAW in my travel analogy is this: If you are very rich and have lots of free time, you don't really have to plan your vacations that carefully. You can wait until the last minute and almost always get a flight out and a place to stay.

That's not always true in Malady. Sure, being rich and well-connected can help get you to a top doctor at a major treatment center, as well as pay for a private room in the deluxe wing and a suite in a nearby hotel for the family.

But, be you a Rockefeller or just a fella, if you wait too long, and fail to do your research, take precautions, and stay alert, you'll be dead before you know it.

As best you can, take charge of your journey.

Acknowledgments

Theron Raines, my friend and agent for more than thirty-five years, and Jonathan Segal, my friend and editor for more than twenty years, were the godfathers and midwives of this book, calling it into being and shaping it along the way. I am grateful beyond this page.

Most of the people who were important to the writing of this book were important to me, period. They were as critical to my healing as they were to my prose.

There were nurses who became friends: Renee S. Trambert, Maryellen O'Sullivan, and Susan Alfano.

There were doctors who became friends: Tom Reynolds, Davor Vugrin, and Paul Russo.

There were friends who happened to be doctors: Mark Chapman, Arthur Rifkin, Paul Stolley, Elizabeth Beautyman, Keith Reemstma, Gordon Potts, and Dave Kinne, who at every treacherous turn on the roads of Malady has been there with kindness, advice, and scalpel.

Carolyn and Joe Lelyveld have been steadfast friends for thirty years. Roger Sims, Michael Forester, Jane Heller, Neal Conan, Janet Roach, Jonathan Kandell, Karen DeCrow, Maria Glaser, Susan B. Adams, and Sari Feldman have always had encouraging words. Carey Winfrey, who invented my "Close Encounters" column for *American Health* magazine, helped me find my voice for this book. Dave Smith, Paul Fishleder, and Joan Nassivera, editors of the *New York Times*

"City Weekly" section, helped me refine that voice in the "Coping" column.

And then there's the *Times*'s sports editor, Neil Amdur, my friend and coach and spiritual advisor.

In sickness and in health, my sister, Gale, and my parents, Fanny and Sidney Lipsyte, have been my safe havens. My wife, Kathy Sulkes, along with everything else she gives me, also gave the understanding and the psychic space to be with Margie in person and in memory.

I hope this book is a proper memorial to Margie and, more important, reflects what she had in mind when she so generously shared her thoughts and her notes for it. She was my best editor.

Thanking Sam and Susannah is like thanking the Sun. They are the light and the warmth of this journey, and of my life.

A Note About the Author

ROBERT LIPSYTE is a sports and city columnist for the *New York Times*. In 1966 and in 1996, he won Columbia University's Mike Berger Award for distinguished reporting. In 1992, he was a finalist for the Pulitzer Prize for commentary. His books include the best-selling Young Adult novel *The Contender* and *SportsWorld: An American Dreamland*. Lipsyte has also been a correspondent for CBS's "Sunday Morning with Charles Kuralt," and for NBC News. In 1990, he won an Emmy for on-camera achievement as host of "The Eleventh Hour," a nightly public affairs program on New York's PBS Channel 13. He lives in Manhattan with his wife.

A Note on the Type

The text of this book was set in Sabon, a typeface designed by Jan Tschichold (1902–1974), the well-known German typographer. Based loosely on the original designs by Claude Garamond (c. 1480–1561), Sabon is unique in that it was explicitly designed for hot-metal composition on both the Monotype and Linotype machines as well as for film-setting. Designed in 1966 in Frankfurt, Sabon was named for the famous Lyons punch cutter Jacques Sabon, who is thought to have brought some of Garamond's matrices to Frankfurt.

Composed by North Market Street Graphics,
Lancaster, Pennsylvania
Printed and bound by
R. R. Donnelley & Sons,
Harrisonburg, Virginia
Designed by Virginia Tan